BEAT SUGAR ADDICTION NOW!

The Cutting[...] [...] That Gets Your Kids Off Sugar Safely, Easily, and Without Fights and Drama

FOR KIDS

JACOB TEITELBAUM, M.D.
Best Selling Author of *Beat Sugar Addiction Now!*

DEBORAH KENNEDY, PH.D.
Founder and CEO, Build Healthy Kids

FAIR WINDS
PRESS

First published in the USA in 2012 by Fair Winds Press, a member of
Quayside Publishing Group
100 Cummings Center, Suite 406-L Beverly, MA 01915-6101
www.fairwindspress.com

16 15 14 13 12   1 2 3 4 5

ISBN: 978-1-59233-523-7

Digital edition published in 2012
eISBN-13: 9-781-61058-618-4

Library of Congress Cataloging-in-Publication Data
Teitelbaum, Jacob.
  Beat sugar addiction now! for kids : the cutting-edge program that gets kids off sugar safely, easily, and without
fights and drama / Jacob Teitelbaum and Deborah Kennedy.
      p. cm.
  Includes index.
  Summary: "The modern American child's diet is awash in sugar–including mainstays such as juice, chocolate milk,
sugary cereals, soda, energy drinks, and fast-food burgers and nuggets with added corn syrup and sweeteners,
let alone candy and cookies prevalent at school parties and play dates. Beat Sugar Addiction Now! for Kids gives
parents a proven 5-step plan for getting and keeping their child off sugar. Bestselling author and noted physician
Dr. Jacob Teitelbaum and pediatric nutrition specialist Deborah Kennedy, Ph.D., give parents a toolkit for avoiding
the common pitfalls such as guilt and temper tantrums, managing the 5-step process successfully on a day-to-day
basis, and getting their child emotionally, as well as physically, unhooked from sugary drinks, breakfast foods,
snacks, and desserts, as well as "hidden" sugars in foods"– Provided by publisher.
  ISBN 978-1-59233-523-7 (pbk.)
  1. Sugar-free diet. 2. Sugar–Physiological effect. 3. Children–Nutrition–Psychological aspects. 4. Health.
I. Kennedy, Deborah. II. Title.
  RM237.85.T45 2012
  613.2'8332–dc23

                                                                                    2012006185

Book design by Kathie Alexander

Printed and bound in U.S.A.

*The information in this book is for educational purposes only. It is not intended to replace the advice of a physician or
medical practitioner. Please see your health care provider before beginning any new health program.*

Dedication

JT: To Laurie, my wife, my best friend, and the love of my life, and to my son, Dave, daughters Amy, Shannon, Brittany, and Kelly, and grandkids Payton and Bryce, who seem to have been born knowing what I'm just learning.

DK: To the three loves of my life: Michael, Kyle, and Bryan. My boys are a constant reminder to me that our health comes down to the choices we make each and every day we walk on this beautiful planet.

Contents

Introduction

Does your children's day with food look something like this: juice and cereal, a doughnut or a toaster cake for breakfast; chocolate milk, a peanut butter and jelly sandwich, and a granola bar for lunch; soda or a juice box with cookies after school; and white pasta with spaghetti sauce, no vegetables, and dessert for dinner? If so, they most likely are addicted to sugar or, at the very least, strongly prefer sweet-tasting processed items to such a degree that they eat small amounts, if any, of the whole grains, vegetables, and protein they need to grow up healthy and strong.

Some of you know for sure that your child is addicted to sugar; some of you may think that your child has an issue with eating too much sugar but are not sure whether you would call him or her an addict. This book applies to either situation, especially if any of the following are true for your child.

- Your child drinks more than one sweet beverage a day (including juice, soda, flavored milk, sports and energy drinks, flavored water, sweetened teas or coffee) *Or*
- Your child's breakfast usually centers on something sweet, such as sugar-sweetened cereal, a doughnut, a toaster cake, a breakfast bar, pancakes, or waffles *Or*
- Your child eats more than one or two sweet treats a day (candy, cookies, pies, yogurt sticks, fruit roll-ups or gummy fruit, cake, cupcakes, or frozen desserts like ice cream) *Or*
- Your child eats little for dinner (and may eat few to no vegetables) but always has room for a sweet dessert *Or*
- Your child has trouble stopping at one serving of a sweet food and screams for more *Or*
- Your child's mood seems to be determined by diet; he or she gets full of energy after a sweet treat and crashes an hour or two later

You have picked up this book because you have a child who consumes lots of items high in sugar. The good news is that by following the steps in this book, you will be able to reverse his or her preference for highly sweetened foods.

Are you ready now to start your children on a five-step journey toward turning their sugar addiction around? We hope so. We have, between us seven, children and more than fifty years of experience in dealing with children and their diets.

We developed this step-by-step program with these essential elements:

1. Easy to follow. Your child focuses on making just one change at a time until he or she reaches the goal. You can follow the steps in the order they are presented or jump to whichever step you determine is most important.

2. Easy on your child. We take it slowly to lessen and limit the negative side effects on your child that often occur when reducing sugar intake. It took your child a long time to develop these unhealthy eating habits, and we allow for as much time as is necessary to turn them around.

3. Easier for you. We give you enough information, tools, and practical advice to make sure that your child follows the program. At the end of the day, getting your child on board is essential for turning around his or her sugar addiction.

Convincing Your Child

What is the harm in giving your children a couple of cookies every day? None. We are not here to completely eliminate sweets from your children's diet; rather, we invite you to limit the amount of added sugar they consume in a day. In most cases, that cookie is not the only source of added sugar in a typical day. They most likely start off with a sugar-laden breakfast, drink chocolate milk, juice boxes, or soda throughout the day, grab a granola bar or fruit gummies as a snack, and eat dessert after dinner.

These added sugar sources add up to increased risks of your child becoming overweight or obese and developing diabetes, heart disease, certain cancers, and behavioral and learning disorders. In addition, they may get more cavities, build softer bones, which may lead to osteoporosis and fractures, and develop a weakened immune system. The hard truth is that allowing your children to eat an unhealthy diet with lots of added sugar means they may not reach their full potential for growth and intelligence or develop a strong immune system. Those are high stakes!

Sometimes, it helps to put these potential consequences in terms that are more real to children who normally (and healthfully) feel immortal. Examples include:

- Research has shown that a low-sugar, high-protein diet cut acne by half after 12 weeks. The good news? Chocolate did not worsen the acne.
- A high intake of sugar was associated with a dramatic increase in bone fractures in children.
- High sugar intake results in nutritional deficiencies that not only leave children less able to compete in sports or school, but also may cause a delay in sexual maturation during puberty.

Twenty-Three Spoonfuls of Sugar a Day

Our kids consume 28 percent more sugar than they did only sixteen years ago, and this rate is rising. In the U.S. Department of Agriculture's (USDA) *Dietary Guidelines for Americans, 2010*, based on data from 2003 and 2004, American children averaged about 23 teaspoons (92 g) of sugar a day, or 175 cups

> The U.S. Department of Agriculture advises limiting the amount of added sugar to no more than 8 teaspoons (32 g) a day in a 2,000-calorie diet. Our kids are getting double to almost triple that amount.

(35 kg) a year! Twenty-three teaspoons (92 g) of added sugar a day equals about 78 pounds (35 kg) a year, which is equal to the average weight of a nine-year-old girl. Many younger children consume their weight, or more, in added sugar every year!

To put it in perspective, the USDA advises limiting the amount of added sugar and total fat calories to no more than 260 calories a day, which would translate to about 8 teaspoons (32 g) a day of added sugar in a 2,000-calorie diet, with half the remaining calories being reserved for solid fats. Our kids are getting double to almost triple that amount—and this is a conservative estimate. Data suggests that children are not the only ones consuming too much sugar. The average adult consumes 140 to 150 pounds (64 to 68 kg) of sugar added to their diet each year from processed food and beverages.

To determine your child's average daily consumption of added sugar, go to the "sugar calculator" on www.BuildHealthyKids.com. Here, you can input the amount of food and beverages your child commonly consumes and get a readout of how much that equals over a year's time. We have also provided a sugar tracking sheet at the end of chapter 1.

Average Added Sugar Intake in Kids' Diets During 2003–2004

Age	Added sugar Kcal/per day	Added sugar per year	Added sugar per year
2 to 3 years	197	94 cups (19 kg)	42 lbs (19 kg)
4 to 8 years	329	156 cups (31 kg)	69 lbs (31 kg)
9 to 13 years	381	181 cups (36 kg)	80 lbs (36 kg)
14 to 18 years	444	211 cups (42 kg)	94 lbs (42 kg)

Source: National Cancer Institute

The 23 teaspoons (92 g) a day of added sugar does not include sugar in its natural form, like that found in fruit, grains, or milk products. It includes white sugar, brown sugar, corn syrup, corn syrup solids, raw sugar, malt syrup, maple syrup, pancake syrup, fructose sweetener, liquid fructose, honey, molasses, anhydrous dextrose, high-fructose corn syrup (which manufacturers may change to "corn syrup" because it has received such a bad rap), and crystal dextrose.

Where are our kids getting most of these sugars from? The answer is found in the following table. The top three sources of added sugar in our children's diets are soda, fruit drinks, and grain-based desserts (cake, cookies, pie, cobbler, sweet rolls, pastries, and doughnuts).

Sources of Added Sugar in the Diets of
American Children and Adolescents, 2003–2004

Rank	Food item	Percent contribution
1	Soda, energy and sports drinks	31.8 percent
2	Fruit drinks	15.0 percent
3	Grain-based desserts	10.9 percent
4	Dairy desserts	7.9 percent
5	Candy	6.8 percent
6	Ready-to-eat cereal	6.4 percent
7	Syrups/toppings	2.8 percent
8	Tea	2.1 percent
9	Yeast breads	1.9 percent
10	Whole milk	1.7 percent

Source: National Cancer Institute

Negative Effects Associated with Eating a Diet High in Sugar

Studies have shown that children who eat a diet high in sugar are more at risk for the following:

- Attention deficit and hyperactivity disorder and other learning and behavioral disorders
- Anxiety and depression
- Bone fractures
- Cavities
- Candida (yeast)
- Chronic fatigue syndrome and fibromyalgia
- Chronic sinusitis and ear infections
- Decreased immune function, and increased susceptability to infections and serious diseases like cancer
- Diabetes
- Heart disease
- Irritable bowel syndrome and spastic colon (which accounts for 50 percent of abdominal pains)
- Metabolic syndrome

The Roller-Coaster Ride of Sugar and Insulin

If you wonder how sugar can affect so many aspects of health, let us explain. When children eat sugar, their blood sugar level rises. How much depends on what type of sugar they ate and what else they ate with the sugar. For example, eating a piece of fruit that has fiber in it will cause less of a rise in blood sugar than ingesting a lollipop, juice, or soda, which is just straight sugar. Also, if your child eats protein or fat along with sugar, her blood sugar level will not rise as quickly or as high compared to if she ate sugar alone.

As blood sugar levels rise, your child's pancreas releases insulin, which is the key that lets sugar into the cells so that it can provide energy. If there is no insulin or just not enough insulin around (called insulin resistance or in type 1 diabetes) or the insulin stopped letting the sugar into the cells (as in type 2 diabetes), your child's blood sugar level rises beyond the normal range, and this is when a lot of damage can happen. The body tightly regulates blood sugar levels because extra sugar in the blood can damage the kidneys, eyes, blood vessels, and just about everything else. It is not healthy to have a level of sugar in the blood that is either too low (hypoglycemia) or too high (diabetes).

Several factors increase your child's chances of developing type 2 diabetes: being overweight and not exercising are the top two, but having an unhealthy eating pattern that includes too much fat and/or sugar also puts your child at risk. Beverages and foods with a lot of added sugar constantly require your child's pancreas to pump out insulin. Over time, the pancreas can become exhausted and not do a good job releasing enough insulin that the cells need, or the cells themselves can become resistant to letting the sugar in, which is what you see with obesity. Are our kids eating the amount of sugar that will cause their pancreas to say "enough" or will make them gain so much weight that their cells become resistant? You bet. Type 2 diabetes is on the rise.

Beat Sugar Addiction Now for Kids

Children born today have a one in three chance of developing diabetes in their lifetime, and this goes up to a one in two chance if they are African American or Hispanic. The result of insulin resistance is far reaching. In individuals who have insulin resistance, sugar raises their levels of triglycerides, which can lead to heart disease.

Sugar can drive your child's immune system into both underfunction and overdrive, with neither working to your child's advantage. Research has shown that the function of white blood cells, called macrophages, which patrol the body to prevent outside invasion, is decreased by more than 30 percent for three hours after consuming the amount of sugar in a can of soda. Meanwhile, other parts of the immune system that regulate inflammation are put into overdrive, increasing the risk of autoimmune conditions. This can occur from exhausting the immune-modulating adrenal hormones as well as from immune deficiencies (especially of inflammation-calming omega-3 oils) caused by sugar's empty calories.

When children eat and drink so much sugar in lieu of eating a well-balanced diet, they don't get enough of the nutrients they need for optimal health and growth, such as fiber, vitamins A, C, and E, and folate, magnesium, and calcium. Children replace milk, the number one source of calcium in their diet, with soft drinks. Because of this, their intake of the calcium needed to build bones is insufficient, which can lead to softer bone development and result in fractures and osteoporosis. It is also likely that the minerals in their bones are lost to buffer the high acidity in sodas, which also leads to softer bones.

Sugar can cause behavioral havoc, with both immediate and long-term consequences. For example, most parents are familiar with the effects of rapid shifts in blood sugar that occur after eating a lot of sugar: kids initially run on overdrive for a few hours, then become irritable, and finally, drop into couch potato mode. These behaviors correspond to an initial spike in sugar (the high),

> Low blood sugar triggers the same signals as suffocation: a heavy adrenaline release followed by irritability and sugar-craving behavior.

followed by irritability as the body senses blood sugar dropping, and then fatigue when the blood sugar is low.

This doesn't occur with whole foods because the body absorbs sugars in these foods over two to three hours, causing a mild rise in blood sugar. The body is designed to read that rise in sugar and put out just enough insulin to carry the sugar from the blood into your cells. It presumes that the sugar will continue to be coming into the blood over three hours as the food digests.

With processed sugars, however, it all gets absorbed into the bloodstream in minutes. The body sees this sugar spike and presumes you ate a massive amount, so it pours out insulin, enough for its usual two to three hours. An hour later, the sugar is gone but the insulin is still pouring out, driving blood sugar way down. The low blood sugar triggers the same signals as suffocation: a heavy adrenaline release followed by irritability and sugar-craving behavior. If your child then eats more sugar, the pattern repeats, sending him or her on an emotional sugar roller-coaster ride. If not, your child's energy crashes.

The long-term problems can be even more severe: nutritional deficiencies, and the social impact of the short-term behavioral problems, catch up with the child. A new study suggests that a high sugar intake poses a danger not only to the child but also to others around him. Specifically, in a large survey of Boston high school students, those who drank more soda (five or more cans per week) were markedly more likely to act violently toward peers, siblings, and people they were dating. They were also much more likely to carry weapons.

A frightening thought? Drinking soda, even one can a day, was as likely to be associated with student violence as underage drinking and smoking. And the more soda the children drank, the more violent they became. This suggests that even moderate cutbacks in soda intake can make a big difference.

Developing a Taste for Processed Food

We have never seen a child eat too much fruit, vegetables, or whole grains in our practices, but we have seen many who consume a lot of juice, soda, candy, doughnuts, cookies, and other highly processed items. You have probably observed the same with your children.

Did you ever wonder why that is? Most likely this preference for processed foods started when food became engineered in a laboratory instead of baked in a kitchen or picked in a field. Once food became highly processed and food scientists entered the picture, food went from, to put it simply, a *food* to a *drug* for some. Scientists refer to these highly processed foods as hyperpalatable—they taste super yummy. They are sweeter, saltier, and fattier than most foods found in nature, so they fool your taste buds. Foods found in nature can't compete with processed foods for the same taste satisfaction.

When children start to eat solid food, they love fruits and vegetables, legumes, and the straight-from-nature foods. It is only when they are exposed to these highly sweet, savory, and salty tastes that they develop a preference for foods and beverages high in these tastes. This preference for artificially sweet-tasting food is learned, which is a good thing, because it means it can be unlearned.

No one is immune to becoming addicted to sugar because we are all born preferring a sweet taste, which has been shown to soothe us even in infancy.

Imagine that babies' tongues are blank canvases that will be painted on with different tastes from the foods they are given as they age. What you feed them over and over again is what they learn to like: give them vegetables and they will learn to like vegetables; allow them to eat lots of sugary food and they will prefer sweet items. This also applies to older children and adults. If you eat a diet high in sugar, you get used to that super-sweet taste and, therefore, "need" a high sugar taste to be satisfied. Once you reduce your intake of sugar, your taste buds will reacclimate to a preference for a natural (less) sweet taste.

Research is finally supporting what many nutritionists and psychologists have known for years: food can be addictive, especially sweet-tasting foods and drinks. Twenty-eight scientific studies and papers on food addiction were published in the first ten months of 2011 alone.

"The data is so overwhelming, the field has to accept it," said Nora Volkow, director of the National Institute on Drug Abuse. "We are finding tremendous overlap between drugs in the brain and food in the brain."

There are many similarities between hyperpalatable foods (which include foods high in sugar) and addictive drugs on eating behavior and the brain's response to sweets. Studies that looked at the brain found similar responses in certain areas between those addicted to food and those addicted to drugs and alcohol. There are also many studies in the animal literature supporting the addictive quality of sugar.

Who is susceptible to this addiction? Those with a family history of addiction are susceptible, but no one is immune to becoming addicted to sugar because we are all born preferring a sweet taste, which has been shown to soothe us even in infancy. Even if your family history does not include addiction, your children can still develop a problem with sugar. Whether or not they can be technically classified as having an addiction is not really the issue. If your children's diet consists of so much added sugar that they are not eating the healthy nutrients they need to grow up big and strong, then their sugar intake is a problem.

The creation of these hyperpalatable foods have made it extremely difficult for parents to put limits on their children's intake of sugar. Before the industrial revolution, we would have cake when mom took the time to bake it herself. If it wasn't there, we didn't have hundreds of other items to choose from at the store, or our friend's house, or in school. Nowadays, even if we take the time to prepare a great healthy meal for our children, they often refuse to eat it because they prefer the taste of processed items instead. Most of us have heard the excuse "I'm full" at the dinner table only to hear screams of hunger for dessert, crackers, chips, or ice cream minutes later.

If you follow the advice of your child's pediatrician and most dieticians, you are told not to insist, push, or even encourage your children to eat. You are told that any interference from you will have negative consequences and that it is your job to decide *where* your children will eat and *what* to feed them, and it is your children's job to decide *whether* they want to eat and *how much* they want to eat. That sounds like good advice, but in the real world it has disempowered a generation or two of parents, who are told to back off at the kitchen table.

> *If we, as parents, cannot encourage or enforce rules at the dinner table, then we have lost the battle before it has even started, and our kids will pay the price with their health.*

Kids learn to play this system of *what* and *where/whether* and *how much* with ease and often refuse to eat what is in front of them and insist on only eating what they want to eat later on. Most times what they want are not the healthy vegetables and whole grains but processed white flour and added-sugar items. This advice gives children's taste buds free rein, leading them down a path where a large chunk of their diet comes from white processed foods high in sugar, with the majority not meeting their daily requirements for vegetables, fiber, and calcium.

Eating is a behavior that we teach our children like any other—healthy sleep habits, getting along with others, good hygiene. How many of our kids would voluntarily put themselves to bed because we told them to once and then backed off? If we were not permitted to enforce or encourage them to get to bed on time, not many would. The same holds true for eating. If we as parents cannot encourage or enforce rules at the dinner table, then we have lost the battle before it has even started, and our kids will pay the price with their health.

It doesn't need to be a power struggle, though. Rights naturally come with responsibilities. Certain privileges (the amount of their allowance, being able to go to a movie or a friend's house, getting to stay up sometimes for "special nights," getting a special toy or even a cell phone or phone minutes) come with certain actions (such as getting good grades, eating healthfully, and so on).

We are giving you permission to set rules and consequences at the dinner table. We are asking you to use methods that are tried and true over the eons for most behaviors that we want to encourage in our children. Take back your power. It is time to teach this generation of children how to follow a healthy diet. You will receive tips and tools throughout the five steps in this book to help you do just that. Encouragement, setting rules, enforcing consequences, and especially out-and-out bribery are all allowed. Let's begin!

Chapter 1

Getting Started:
The Parent Tool Kit for
Ensuring Success

How to minimize the fights, tears, and drama that can come from taking away your children's favorite treats

You have picked up this book and you are pumped and ready to take your child off of added sugar. The only problem is, your children will most likely not feel the same way. They may resist your efforts and kick and scream each step of the way. So we've created this parent tool kit to help you get your children on your side. In addition, we offer tips and advice throughout the book to help your child succeed.

For very young children, you may be able to avoid getting them actively involved. Younger children may not notice when you substitute healthy drinks for the unhealthy ones, switch to more wholesome snacks and meals, and buy products with limited added sugar. For preschoolers, you still have some control over what they eat and can make some healthy changes without them knowing, but you still need their cooperation and commitment to a degree. Teens and tweens will need to know why they should follow the program and what it entails each step of the way. Having them agree to be part of the process on a voluntary basis is very important. If they are not on board, removing added sugar from their diet will not be successful. They will just become sneakier about eating and drinking products high in sugar when you are not around.

> Removing all sugar from your child's diet at once leads to tantrums and outbursts, plus major withdrawal symptoms.

Getting your children to partner with you entails having them understand the need for cutting back on sugar and offering rewards for doing so. We want to be rewarded for the work we do (e.g., earning a paycheck), and so do our children. Agree on certain rewards they will receive for success at different points during the process—and make them valuable enough to leave your child motivated. It'll be a great investment!

Parents often ask how long it will take for children to kick their addiction. We cannot give you a solid answer because it depends on your child's level of addiction, the stress level in her life, her personality, and your commitment and involvement in the process. The prescriptions in each chapter give you one month to make a major shift in your child's intake of sugar. It may, at most, take 5 months, but it could take fewer months if your child doesn't need to follow each step.

As much as we would have liked to make it a speedy process in reversing your child's addiction to sugar, we do not want to compromise your child's long-term success in adhering to a low-sugar diet. Our step-by-step program design in *Beat Sugar Addiction Now for Kids* was intentional because a quick change is not in your or your child's best interest. Removing all sugar from your child's diet at once leads to tantrums and outbursts, plus major withdrawal symptoms. Instead, we have designed this program so as not to disrupt your child's life too much, which will significantly limit any major kickback from your kids. We built in enough time during each step to set new, healthier habits, thus limiting the risk that your child will quickly fall back to her "sugar ways."

Getting Started

Throughout this book, we provide plenty of information to teach and motivate your child. At the end of the day, knowing that your children have the information and motivation to make healthy choices on their own is really what it is all about.

Below are age-appropriate instructions for discussing with your children why you are removing most of the added sugar from their diet and how you are going to do it. For each group, start by calculating their daily sugar intake by using the "Daily Added Sugar Tracking Tool" at the end of the chapter.

• **TWO-YEAR-OLDS**

Parents have total control over the diet of children this age, and two-year-olds don't have the cognitive ability to understand what you are doing and why you are doing it. Instead, they just know that their juice tastes different or they can no longer have a cookie. It is best with this age group to simply avoid explanations.

Young children don't have the long-term exposure to eating food with added sugar that older children would have, but drinking lots of sugary beverages may be all that they know. Replacing unhealthy choices with healthy ones, and doing it gradually, will be the best method for working with children of this age. Your goal as the parent is to make the changes slowly so as not to disrupt their lives too much.

You most likely will get some pushback from them during this program, and when this occurs, we recommend you distract them as you would in other situations. When they scream for the cookie, for example, offer fruit instead, and pull out their favorite book to read, or go out to play. If you keep their mind off of the fact that they cannot have their cookie, they may soon forget about it. If they don't and pitch a tantrum, allow them the space to have their tantrum. If you give in, they learn that a tantrum gets them what they want and they will continue to use this behavior in the future to get their way.

✔ Summary

☐ Start by calculating their daily sugar consumption.

☐ Avoid explanations.

☐ Switch to healthier products.

☐ Reduce sugar-laden foods and drinks gradually.

☐ Distract them when they want sweets.

- **PRESCHOOL-AGE CHILDREN**

Three-, four-, and five-year-olds will notice and question why they cannot have their third juice box or the pudding pop they are used to eating for an afternoon snack. They most likely have a routine that they are used to: sweet cereal for breakfast, gummy fruit for snack, and dessert at lunch.

They will need some explanation when you remove their favorites from their diet, but keep it as brief as possible. Do not draw their attention to when you switch foods. If they do notice, let them know that you are buying healthy food and not junk food. Teaching them the difference between food that is healthy and food that is not is the main focus for preschoolers. Keep repeating that healthy food makes them "grow up big and strong" like their daddy, mommy, or another favorite adult, and junk food is a treat they can have occasionally, but it doesn't make them healthy.

Use a Point System to Motivate Children

A point system can be your biggest ally during this program. With this system, children earn points or stickers for each step that they successfully complete.

The point system works well for children in second grade and above, while stickers work just fine for younger kids (usually children younger than five or six). Depending on the age of the child, just getting a sticker is motivation enough. For the older child, accumulating points that go toward receiving a prize or gift at the end is a huge motivating factor for them to stick with the program, as long as the prize is something that they really want.

We have included a pledge at the end of this chapter for you and your child to sign that lists the prizes that he or she will earn after making the necessary changes. (See "Beat Sugar Addiction Pledge.")

Children in this age group are motivated to be just like the "bigger" people in their life. They will not understand specific health risks, but they do understand the concept of growing and getting big. The younger child needs less technical explanations: "We don't drink that anymore" and "That is a treat and it doesn't make us grow up big and strong" are reason enough for this age group. Keep your language inclusive, for all ages, because the more you include yourself, the less alienating it will be for your child. For example, say, "We don't eat this" as opposed to "You can't eat this."

Do not focus on weight when talking to children because it may not be an accurate predictor of their health and it may lead to an unhealthy obsession about weight. Use words like healthy or unhealthy, strong or weak, fast or slow, and tall or not reaching your potential height instead of words that focus on their weight, like fat, obese, overweight, or chunky.

When times get rough and they are screaming for a sweet food or drink, distract them by doing something together. Sometimes, children are looking for a connection and reach out to junk food to feel good. Spend time connecting with them instead of backing away when things get tough—play a game, ride bikes together, or color or paint, for example. If this doesn't work, give them space in their own room to work it out.

✔ Summary

☐ Start by calculating their daily sugar consumption.

☐ Teach them the difference between junk food and healthy food.

☐ Use words and phrases such as "growing up big and strong" like their favorite adult as an incentive.

☐ Use inclusive language such as "We don't eat this way."

☐ Distract and connect.

☐ Create a point or sticker system beginning at this age.

- **ELEMENTARY SCHOOL–AGED CHILDREN (FIRST THROUGH SIXTH GRADE)**

  Food habits are deeply engrained in children six to eleven years of age. They are also old enough to understand the health consequences of their actions, especially if these consequences are presented to them in a personal manner. For example, let them know that the amount of sugar they eat will affect their stamina and ability to play soccer, or concentrate as long on their studies, or be as strong in martial arts. They can understand that they need healthy food to play their best, and sugar will only cause an initial rush of energy followed by a crash soon afterward.

You can also get their cooperation by presenting the project as a scientific experiment. Engaging this age group with a focus on their bodies is a key element to success. Start by first figuring out their total sugar consumption together. Go to the sugar calculator at www.BuildHealthyKids.com to determine how much sugar they eat or fill in the sugar-tracking sheet at the end of this chapter. Once you have the daily sugar total, discuss with them how eating that amount of sugar will affect what they do every day. Be as specific as you can, and focus on what they love to do best.

To determine how much sugar they consume away from home, do your homework. Many schools have removed soda and sports drinks from vending machines, but some elementary school children can still buy sugar-sweetened beverages and junk food at their schools. Look at your school's health and wellness policy to see whether there are rules prohibiting the sale of junk food, or talk to your child's principal. Review your child's weekly/monthly cafeteria menu together and buy food on days when there are healthy options such as items that are made with whole grains and are low in sugar, not French toast sticks and cereal.

Once you know what is available, you are better prepared to ask your children what they chose for lunch. Start by asking, "What did you drink and eat at lunch today—milk, juice, or water?" (whatever is sold at their school), followed by, "Did you finish your drink?" You can slowly piece together the amount and types of beverages and foods they consumed away from home. Question children in a nonthreatening manner and try to elicit their help.

Once you are armed with the total daily sugar consumption and its negative effects, you are ready to get their cooperation to remove sugary items from their diet. If reviewing the total sugar amounts with its consequences is not enough to convince them to do the program, then let them know that you have decided that they are going to follow the program and list your reasons why. Most children this age still listen to the direction of their parents; they may not like it, but they will do it because mom or dad said so. Let them know what the rules are and what you expect of them during each step of the program. List the consequences of not following those steps: every time they eat or drink a sugary product, they have an increase in chores, lose phone, TV, or computer time for a day, have to pay you $1 to $5 (that you save up and spend on the prize at the end), or anything else that will motivate them to follow the rules.

Most important, though, reward them for their positive steps along the way, while offering them a major prize when they finish the program. The gift or prize can serve as a distraction for your children. They can focus on what they will get as opposed to what has been taken away from them. Consider also a smaller gift at the end of each of the five steps. If you select the right gifts, it will help make following the program that much easier for all of you.

If money is an issue, the gift does not have to cost anything. It can be as simple as a promise that dad will play ball after work every day for a week or mom will spend time with them working on an art project. Sometimes, a great gift is time with mom and dad or their favorite aunt, uncle, or grandparent. Offering them greater rights for having shown greater responsibility is another option. Just make sure you do not offer them a food-related prize, because this would be sending the wrong message.

✔ Summary

- ☐ Calculate your child's total sugar consumption.
- ☐ Focus on sugar's effect on their body.
- ☐ Make consequences personal.
- ☐ Set rules and consequences.
- ☐ Offer a prize.

You do not want to approach tweens or teens with an ultimatum because this will most likely backfire.

• **TWEENS AND TEENS**

For tweens and teens, you will need to sit down and have a discussion with them about why you are concerned about their consumption of added sugar and why you want them to follow this program. It is best with this age group to start by calculating how many grams or spoons of sugar they eat and drink in a day, followed by the consequences of eating that much sugar. You can either have them calculate their daily added sugar amount by themselves or you can do it together, depending on the relationship that you have with your kids.

Be specific when listing the health consequences. Increased sugar intake puts them at increased risk for diabetes, heart disease, becoming overweight or obese, and breaking bones during sports. It makes it harder for them to concentrate on their schoolwork and may aggravate any underlying hyperactivity disorder like ADHD. It also can worsen acne and lead to cavities, as well as the other consequences listed in the beginning of this book and throughout each of the steps.

Focus on the health consequences that have the most significant effect on them. For instance, if they consume energy drinks, have them read the section on the negative effects of energy drinks in chapter 2. Bring in your and your spouse's health history if your child is your biological child. "Grandma had diabetes, but you can prevent it," and "Your dad has high blood pressure and his dad died of heart disease," are examples of conversations that you can have with your teen or tween. They are at an age when they need to know what their genetic health risks are so that they can make decisions based on this information. Let them know that just because their parents or grandparents had a disease, it doesn't mean they will get that disease, too. The decisions they make now and in their future have a huge influence on whether they develop heart disease or diabetes.

You do not want to approach tweens or teens with an ultimatum because this will most likely backfire. Instead, tell them that you really want them to follow this program, explain why, and elicit their help in figuring out what it will take to get them on board. If information about the amount of sugar they are eating plus the consequences of eating it is not enough to sway them, bribery can be a healthy resort. Most, if not all, tweens and teens are motivated to acquire more stuff, such as a new phone or phone plan, computer program, clothes, sneakers, money, and sports equipment. You know your children best and your financial ability to purchase a gift for them. Picking the item they want more than anything goes a long way in buying their cooperation to follow the five-step program.

Once they start to feel better being off the sugar, it will continue to motivate them to stick with the program as well. If you do not have the finances to purchase a prize, be creative and come up with something that does not cost money, such as an extension of their curfew, a sleepover party, time out from chores, a trip to their favorite cousin's house, or more time with their friends.

As a last resort, you can use punishment. If they do not or will not follow the program, take away something that they really care about, such as car privileges, phone time, screen time, or time with their friends, until they are ready to do it. At this age, you really cannot prevent them from eating and drinking what they want away from home, so it is essential that you have their commitment to follow the program.

You will need to enforce rules and consequences throughout the program because most likely, at some point, they will deviate from it and sneak a sweet snack or drink. Have them pay for their decision by doing more chores or taking away their phone for a limited period of time—or you can even consider charging them for it. Each mishap will cost them $5, or whatever cost you think will keep them on the straight and narrow. You can put this money in an account that you give back to them when they go to college; just don't let them know that at the time.

✓ Summary

- ☐ Start by calculating sugar consumption.
- ☐ Voice your concerns.
- ☐ Educate them on their personal health consequences.
- ☐ Develop and explain rules and consequences, bribes and punishment.
- ☐ Offer a prize.

The best thing that you, as a parent, can do is to be consistent and strong throughout the entire program. This is the time that tough love may come into play. Although no one likes to see their children upset or suffering, removing sugar from their diet most likely will upset them. They will go through periods of withdrawal. Know that, in the end, when you have removed added sugar from their diet, it will be worth it. Your children's health and the length of their lives depend on eating a varied, well-balanced diet, and there is little room in that diet for products high in added sugar.

> Seventy-two percent of what kids eat is influenced by their parents.

Once your children are off the sugar completely and have broken their addiction, you will be able to add back in a treat or two. In fact, even during the program they will be allowed one or two treats a day. Research shows that completely forbidding a food causes you to only want more of it.

Making sure that you work with your children, and not against them, is essential for success. You will experience pushback and frustration from your children during this program, but you will be prepared to handle it. We will give you tips and tools throughout the book to make sure that you are equipped to handle most situations.

We have created a prescription to follow to get your child off of sugar-laden drinks and food. Don't be afraid to blame it on us when times get tough: Dr. T and Dr. Deb said that you can't have this because it's not good for you. Depending on the age of your child, you may find that he or she has a bigger issue with one type of food or drink than another. For instance, younger children drink more juice and less soda, whereas older children drink soda and energy drinks and not as much juice, in general. Don't be afraid to tweak the prescription here and there to best suit your children's needs; skip the juice step if your children don't drink any and start with soda if that is where their major issue lies.

How to Get Your Spouse on Board

If we told you that you and your spouse had a major influence on what your children eat, would you believe us? In fact, 72 percent of what kids eat is influenced by their parents. Do you eat a lot of sugar? Do you have a good relationship with food? Children are looking to see what you eat (soda, ice cream, and so on) and how you eat (gobble food, eat distractedly in front of the television) and they imitate you. It is called mirroring, and the scientific literature is clear that your kids will learn a lot from your eating behaviors. As they age, their friends become more of an influence, but what you eat matters, too. They are watching you!

It is important that you and your spouse work together to bring up healthy eaters. If they see one parent eating one way and the other a completely different way, this sets up a situation of confusion for them and creates tension within the family. Are you in a situation where you find yourself fighting against your spouse about what to feed your children? Do you buy healthy food only to find that your husband has come home with a liter of soda or a box of dough-nuts? If you do, you are not alone. We have been asked hundreds of times to intervene between a husband and a wife in these situations. The majority of requests over the years have been moms asking for help with their husbands, with the occasional dad asking for our help.

In these situations, facts and information are essential. Dads don't want to harm their children. More often than not, they are trying to love their children with food. Either they have a special memory about a specific food or drink and want to share that with their children or they just don't realize how unhealthy the food is. Yodels and Ovaltine will always hold special memories for Dr. Deb, but she doesn't buy them for two reasons: She doesn't want to struggle with not eating them herself and she doesn't want to pass down the addiction.

Hard numbers and scientifically backed health consequences speak a thousand words when it comes to getting your spouse on board. The best place

In some cases, parents who sabotage their children's diet are looking for a coconspirator, someone to make them feel less alone or guilty in their own unhealthy eating behavior.

to start the conversation with your seemingly uncooperative spouse is with facts. Begin by determining how much sugar your children consume each day. Then figure out their consumption of added sugar over a year because the impact will be greater. Take, for example, a father whom Dr. Deb worked with who always bought chocolate milk on sale for his son even though his wife asked him not to. When he put ten 5-pound bags of sugar on the kitchen counter—the amount of sugar that his child drank a year in chocolate milk that he bought—he finally realized that buying chocolate milk for his child added up to an insane amount of sugar every year.

The way that you approach your spouse on this issue is the key to success. Most spouses get trapped playing the blame game. It's easy to yell at your spouse and say that your children's unhealthy eating habits are his or her fault. If this technique worked, there would be no need for marriage therapists or counselors. Try sitting down when the two of you are relaxed and ask questions about your spouse's relationship with food. What is he really thinking when he brings home certain foods or drinks? What was dinnertime like when he was growing up? What was her relationship with food like when she was a child? Was she allowed to eat lots of sweet treats? Did he get punished at the dinner table if he didn't eat everything? If this conversation can be done in a casual, friendly manner, you will be more likely to learn the true reasons behind what looks like sabotage to you. And the information that you learn from these conversations is the best place to start. We have made it easy by providing a list of questions at the end of the chapter. (See "Questions for Parents about Their Eating Habits and History.")

In some cases, parents who sabotage their children's diet are looking for a coconspirator, someone to make them feel less alone or guilty in their own unhealthy eating behavior. This is often seen within couples but it also can occur between a parent and a child. The parent bonds with the child over the unhealthy food choice. It is no longer just dad being the "bad guy" because now the tables have turned. Now mom is the "bad guy" who won't let her family eat or drink a specific item. This power struggle is one that needs to be addressed between you and your spouse. Here are five steps to get your spouse on board:

1. Find out the real reason your spouse is buying unhealthy food and beverages or is allowing your child to consume them. Start with an unheated, loving conversation.

2. Determine the daily added sugar total and translate that into a year's worth of added sugar. You can do this for a specific food or for your child's total diet. (Go to the added sugar calculator at www.BuildHealthyKids.com to help determine your child's daily, monthly, and yearly totals.)

3. Show your spouse the list of unhealthy side effects and diseases that can occur from eating a diet too high in sugar.

4. Encourage your spouse to bond with your child over exercise or another activity that isn't food related.

5. Invite your spouse to join the children in beating his or her sugar addiction if this is an issue.

How to Handle Peer Pressure

It was easier years ago to control what our children ate at home during their formative years because if we didn't want them to eat candy, for example, we just wouldn't bring it in the house. As a parent, you didn't need to worry about what other children ate influencing your children's diet for the first five years of their life before you sent them to kindergarten. By the time they entered school, their eating habits were deeply ingrained and you had a fighting chance to bring up your children to eat the diet that you provided.

Today, however, many children join day care at an early age and are thus exposed to many more families' food preferences early on. They see their friend eating cookies or chocolate milk and then they want these sweet items, too.

Peer pressure will influence your children for their entire childhood, especially when they are coming off of sugar. Just as you would not put an alcoholic in the beginning stages of recovery in a room with others who are drinking, you also want to limit the amount of influence that your children's friends have on them, especially during the early stages. Removing sugar-laden foods from your children's diet will not be a "cool thing" socially for your children, so it's best not to share that information with their friends, unless your children choose to disclose it.

Feel free, however, to elicit the help of your children's friends' parents. For younger children, ask their friend's parents not to serve sweet treats like soda or ice cream while your children are on a playdate. Let the parents know what you are doing and why, if you are comfortable with that. Try this: "For health reasons, I have decided to limit sugar in Billy's diet. I could use your help and would really appreciate it if you wouldn't offer him sweet treats during the playdate. I have brought these crackers if you need a snack or he can just have some fruit." Perhaps they will join you on your quest and remove added sugar from their child's diet. Be careful not to push your views on them; stick to the reasons that you are doing it instead of focusing on why their child needs to do

If your child is someone who is easily influenced, be prepared to step in and limit her interaction with children who consume lots of unhealthy food and drinks during the time she is following this program.

it, too. You can also avoid or limit playdates during the early days of recovery if you feel uneasy with others knowing that your child is on the program.

For older children, try to limit the amount of time they spend with friends who consume lots of sugary foods and drinks, at least initially. The only way to do this with older children is to have them on board, understanding why it is important. Setting small, realistic goals will work better than a grand declaration; "Please don't hang out with Nick for the next week" will work far better than "You can't see Nick for the next five months outside of school." Suggest that they hang out in situations that do not require food or drink: bowling and bike rides instead of movies and restaurant outings. Give your children as much information as they need to make the right decisions. In the end, with older children, the decision will be theirs when they are out of your sight. Teach them to view the soda or junk food for what it is: a harmful substance that will affect their long-term health.

During this program, your older child may respond with, "But all my friends drink energy drinks, why can't I?" in a pitch that makes most parents cringe. Respond the same way as you would normally when asked about other things: not wanting to wear a hat when it's cold, dating in middle school, going to the city alone, and so on. We will give you the information to pass along to your children as to why you are making these decisions, and then it is your job as a parent to practice tough love and follow up with "because your health is too important and these drinks are dangerous" repeated as many times as it takes. When all else fails, tell them, "I understand your frustration and I would be frustrated, too. You don't need to like it, you just need to not drink energy drinks (or whatever it is that they are complaining about) because it's for your health."

The amount of intervention that you will need to exert depends on your children's personalities. Some children are followers and others are leaders. You know best which camp your children reside in; they may want to do everything they see their best friend doing, or they do their own thing no matter what. If your child is someone who is easily influenced, be prepared to step in and limit her interaction with children who consume lots of unhealthy food and drinks during the time she is following this program. You do not need to forbid an interaction with a friend that may have a negative influence, just steer the situation to one where food is not involved: a sports outing, a day at the beach, or a trip to the library, for example.

Following the Rules Away from Home

As with any other behavior that we trust our children to follow when they are out of our sight, eating is no different. When we send them out into the world, we hope they will use their manners, get along with others, and not cheat on tests or steal candy from the store. We also hope that when we tell them not to drink soda, especially when they are away from home, that they will follow our rules. If you have not enforced many rules in the past, it may take time for your child to know that you mean business this time. Keeping the rules clear and concise and always enforced will go a long way toward teaching your child that you are serious and that there will be consequences for not following the rules.

If possible, though, especially for older children, it is best to let your children know that you trust them so they will try to live up to your trust—even if they have an occasional lapse. If you simply issue an edict outlawing sugar, it is normal for them to push back and ignore the rules when you are not looking. On the other hand, if children have voluntarily entered an agreement with you, especially to earn a prize, they are much more likely to keep the agreement, because they are then also following their own rules.

Let your children know, especially if you suspect them of lying, that the only ones they are hurting by not following the rules, like drinking soda away from the home, are themselves. Do your homework if you suspect that your child is not telling you the truth or if you cannot get any answer besides "I don't know" when you ask what he ate or drank at school or while in day care. Ask her day care provider whether she ate or drank everything you sent or had any other snack or beverage during the day while under the provider's care. In some school districts, monitoring children's intake of food and drink is easy because parents have access to their child's school cafeteria purchases. If this does not apply to your child's school, look at your child's school cafeteria menu instead. Avoid becoming the "sugar police," though, because this will simply encourage most children to become sneakier and increase sugar intake as a statement of their own freedom. Find a way to make it a joint collaboration. Once it's turned into a power struggle, you've both lost.

Now that you have prepared your spouse and your child, you are ready to begin the five-step process of removing highly sugared foods and beverages from your child's diet. If you have more than one child, make sure everyone follows the same rules. Limiting sugar is important not only for children who are addicted to sugar but also for every child. Children need to have limits on their intake of sugar to be and remain healthy.

Beat Sugar Addiction Pledge

After determining the amount of added sugar in your children's diet, sit down with them and select an age-appropriate prize that they will earn after successfully completing each step. For younger children, attach a picture of what the prize looks like and for older children, have them write down what it will be.

I, _____, promise that I will do my best to follow this program. I understand that too much sugar is not healthy for me.

By following the BSAN for Kids program, I will earn the following:

After Step 1: Eliminate soda, energy drinks, coffee, and caffeinated tea; limit juice; and replace flavored milk, flavored water, and sports drinks with plain milk and water,

I earn: _____

After Step 2: Replace sugary breakfast cereal and avoid pastries, Pop Tarts, and doughnuts, and eat whole grains, whole fruit, and protein at breakfast,

I earn _____

After Step 3: Limit sweet treats to one a day,

I earn _____

After Step 4: Separate dessert from dinner and limit a special dessert to once a week,

I earn _____

After Step 5: Stop the sweet dipping and replace hidden sugars in food with healthy substitutes,

I earn _____

After I finish the program, I agree to keep up the great changes that I have made and

I earn _____

_____   _____
Signature of child   Signature of parent

Questions for Parents about Their Eating Habits and History

Take some time out of your busy schedules to sit down with your partner or spouse. Come together when things are not charged between the two of you and ask each other the following questions. Each partner answers each question before moving on to the next. Take turns going first. Let your partner talk without getting upset, as this is a time when anything goes. Each of your jobs is to just listen and give the other the space to really be heard without judgment. At the end of the conversation you both will decide whether following the program is right for your children.

- What was dinner time like for you growing up? Was everyone there? Was it pleasant, stressful, etc.?
- Did your parents have rules at dinner, and if so, what were they? For example, did you have to clean your plate? What would happen if you didn't follow the rules?
- Did you have to finish your vegetables before getting dessert?
- Did you celebrate with food, such as after getting good grades or winning a game? What was your favorite celebratory treat?
- When you were sick, did your parents use candy to make you feel better?
- Did you eat a lot of sugar growing up? If so what was your favorite sweet? What feeling does it bring up for you?
- Were you able to eat sugar anytime you wanted?
- Do you think that you have an issue with eating too much sugar? If yes, would you like to do something about it?
- Do you think the way you were brought up around food was healthy? Is it something that you want to pass on to your children?
- Which rules, traditions, or structures surrounding food do you want to keep and which ones do you want to throw out?

After learning about your significant other's relationship with food, you both will be in a better place to decide the best strategy for your family. Ask each other whether you both can support the changes that need to be made for your children to follow the *Beat Sugar Addiction Now for Kids* program. It is best if you both could commit to following the steps outlined in program together, but if this is not possible at this time, then at least agree to eat any sweets away from your children during the program.

Daily Added Sugar Tracking Tool

The following calculation will give you a ballpark figure for the grams of added sugar that your children consume in a typical day. For a more accurate measurement, go to www.BuildHealthyKids.com where you will find a sugar calculator. Look at the Nutrition Facts label the food or beverage container for the amount of sugars and serving size.

1. Look at the beverages your children drink and add up the amount they typically drink in a day. Look at the nutrition facts label on the bottle and put in the amount of sugars for

Nutrition Facts	
Serving Size 1 cup (228g)	
Servings Per Container about 2	**Serving Size**
Amount Per Serving	
Calories 250 Calories From Fat 110	
	% Daily Value*
Total Fat 12g	**18%**
Saturated Fat 3g	**15%**
Trans Fat	
Cholesterol 30mg	**10%**
Sodium 470mg	**20%**
Total Carbohydrate 31g	**10%**
Dietary Fiber 0g	**0%**
Sugars 5g	**Sugars**
Proteins 5g	
Vitamin A	**4%**
Vitamin C	**2%**
Calcium	**20%**
Iron	**4%**

Percent Daily Values are based on a 2,000 calorie diet. Your daily values may be higher or lower depending on your calorie needs:

	Calories:	2,000	2,500
Total Fat	Less than	65g	80g
Sat Fat	Less than	20g	25g
Cholesterol	Less than	300mg	300mg
Sodium	Less than	2,400mg	2,400mg
Total Carbohydrate		300g	375g
Dietary Fiber		25g	30g

    a. Soda:

        Grams of sugars per serving _____ × number of servings _____

        = _____ grams of sugar from soda

    b. Flavored milk:

        Grams of sugars per 8 oz serving _____ minus 12 grams *(lactose sugar in 8 oz regular, unflavored milk)* × number of servings _____

        = _____ grams of sugar from flavored milk

    c. Juice:

        Grams of sugars per serving _____ × number of servings *(minus amount your children can have in a day from the number of servings: ages 4 to 6, 6 oz; ages 7 to 13, 8 oz; ages 14 to 18, 12 oz)* = _____ grams of sugar from juice

    d. Energy drinks:

        Grams of sugar per serving _____ × number of servings = _____ grams of sugar from energy drinks

    e. Flavored water:

        Grams of sugar per serving _____ × number of servings = _____ grams of sugar from flavored water

    f. Sports drinks:

        Grams of sugar per serving _____ × number of servings = _____ grams of sugar from sports drinks

    g. Tea and iced tea:

        Grams of sugar per serving _____ × number of servings = _____ grams of sugar from tea and iced tea

    h. Coffee:

        Grams of sugar per serving _____ × number of servings = _____ grams of sugar from coffee

    i. **Total: Add the grams of sugar from each of the beverages above to get a daily total amount of sugars from beverages in your children's diet = _____.**

Daily Added Sugar Tracking Tool (continued)

2. Add up the sugars consumed at breakfast:

    a.   Cereal: _____ grams

    b.   Pop Tarts/doughnuts/pastries: _____ grams

    c.   Pancakes/waffles: _____ grams

    d.   Syrup: number of tablespoons of maple syrup _____ × 12 = _____ grams of sugar

    e.   **Total sugar at breakfast =** _____ **grams**

3. Add up the sugars your children typically eat at lunch time. Look at the Nutrition Facts label to determine grams of sugars per serving. Do not count fruit and unsweetened dairy products.

    a.   For yogurt, multiply grams of sugars by 60 percent: grams of sugars per serving _____ × 0.6 = sugars from yogurt: _____ grams

    b.   Sugars in entrée: _____ grams

    c.   Sugars in dessert: _____ grams

    d.   Bread: If sugar is listed in the ingredient list, take the grams of sugars in bread × 0.93 = _____ grams of sugars in bread (French and Italian bread typically do not have sugar added to the recipe).

    e.   **Total sugar at lunch =** _____ **grams**

4. Add up the sugars your child eats at dinner:

    a.   Dips: _____

    b.   Dessert: _____

    c.   Other: _____

    d.   **Total sugar at dinner =** _____

5. Add up sugars consumed at snack time:

    a.   Morning snack: _____ grams

    For fruit gummies: multiply grams of sugars per serving by 0.66 for grams of sugars in the fruit gummies or fruit bars

    b.   Afternoon snack: _____ grams

    c.   After dinner snack: _____ grams

    For ice cream: multiply grams of sugars in ice cream × 0.86 = _____ sugars in ice cream

    d.   **Totals for sugar from snacks =** _____ **grams**

6. Candy: If you have not already included candy, add that into the calculation now

    a.   Add up the grams of sugars from candy that your child consumes in a typical day:

        _____ total grams

(continued)

Daily Added Sugar Tracking Tool (continued)

7. If you have not already counted the amount of white sugar, brown sugar, honey, or any other sugar, add it in now:

a. Add up teaspoons of white sugar, honey, brown sugar, and other sugars that your children add to their food or drink each day and multiply it by 4 for grams of sugar. _____ teaspoons of added sugar × 4 = total grams of sugar per day _____ from sugar added to food and drink

ADD UP THE SUBTOTALS FROM 1 THROUGH 7 = _____ GRAMS = DAILY SUGAR GRAND TOTAL

Compare your children's daily grand total to their recommended intake:

Age	Added sugar (grams)	Daily sugar grand total
Children 2 to 3	17 grams	#1 _____ grams
Children 4 to 8	15 grams	#2 _____ grams
Boys 9 to 13	20 grams	#3 _____ grams
Boys 14 to 18	33 grams	#4 _____ grams
Girls 9 to 13	15 grams	#5 _____ grams
Girls 14 to 18	20 grams	#6 _____ grams
	GRAND TOTAL:	= _____ **grams**

If your child's daily sugar grand total exceeds the recommended amount, begin the *Beat Sugar Addiction Now for Kids* program as it was designed just for your child!

Daily Added Sugar Tracking Tool (continued)

For shock value, calculate what the daily sugar grand total equals over the course of a year.

DAILY SUGAR GRAND TOTAL _____ **X 365 DAYS =** _____**GRAMS = TOTAL YEARLY CONSUMPTION**

TRANSLATE GRAMS TO CUPS

Total daily grams _____ ÷ 4 = _____ teaspoons

Total teaspoons _____ ÷ 48 = _____ cups

HOW MUCH DOES THAT EQUAL IN 5 LB (2.28 KG) BAGS?

Total cups of sugar _____ ÷ 11.25 = _____ 5 lb (2.28 kg) bags of sugar per year

Chapter 2

Part I

Step 1: How to Limit Liquid Sugar in Your Children's Diet

The skinny on juice, flavored milk, and other "healthy" drinks that your children are hooked on

The first step in your journey toward breaking your children's sugar addiction focuses on dropping their intake of sugar-sweetened beverages. The number one source of added sugar in a child's diet today comes from soda, and energy and sports drinks, according to the USDA's *Dietary Guidelines for Americans, 2010*, which is why the first step in breaking your children's sugar addiction focuses on beverages and not food.

The average child consumes 7½ teaspoons (30 g) of added sugar a day from soda, and energy and sports drinks, and that doesn't take into account the sugar consumed from fruit drinks, flavored milk, and other sugar-sweetened beverages. This may not sound like a lot, but if you calculate what it adds up to in one year, you are looking at 56 cups (11 kg) of added sugar. And that percentage is for the average child. Many consume three to ten times that amount. If this surprises you, consider that sodas have ¾ teaspoon of sugar per ounce. That means that a 48-ounce (1.4 L) "Big Burp" soda from the local Quickie Mart has a whopping 36 teaspoons (144 g) of sugar. It gets scary!

When we consume additional calories from beverages, our body does not compensate for those additional calories by eating less later on.

Until recently in human history we largely drank only water or milk, and most of our nutrients and calories came from food, not beverages. Highly sweetened beverages came on the scene only about 150 years ago, and they were not consumed in any significant amounts until just 50 years ago. Contrast that to today, where the number three source of calories in a child's diet is from beverages. On average, most Americans consume 21 percent of their calories as beverages, and children get 10 to 15 percent of their caloric needs from sugar-sweetened beverages and juice alone. This daily load of sugar is associated with hyperactivity, mood and learning disorders, fatigue, and anxiety, as well as an increased risk for cavities, obesity, prediabetes, type 2 diabetes, and heart disease. If you want to get your teens' attention, let them know that the excess sugar they consume has been shown to be a major cause of acne, as well as zinc deficiency, which can delay their sexual maturation. For a full explanation of the health effects of liquid sugar, see the next section.

One reason for the increase in body weight may be because when we consume additional calories from beverages, our body does not compensate for those additional calories by eating less later on. Our brain will tell our body to eat less at a meal if we ate extra calories from solid food before the meal, but the same is not true if we consumed those same calories from a beverage. Drinking a lot of calories means that children can easily consume too many calories in a day, which leads to weight gain and obesity if it happens over a prolonged period of time. In fact, for the first time in human history, we are seeing high-calorie malnutrition.

How to Begin Limiting Liquid Sugar

Here are the steps for limiting sugared beverages in your children's diet.

1. Figure Out What and How Much Your Children Drink

Begin the process of limiting liquid sugar consumption by first determining how many beverages they consume in a day. This includes everything: water, milk, juice, and sugar-sweetened beverages. Take a day or two to observe how many drinks and what type of beverages they consume. Use the "Daily Beverage Intake Form" provided at the end of the chapter to collect this information. Start each step with the amount of beverages that your child typically con-sumes: for example, if your child drank three juices one day but usually drinks two, start the limiting-juice step by going from two juices a day instead of three. If you are not sure, you can always start with the worst-case scenario, the highest amount that your child drank in a day.

2. Eliminate or Reduce Sweetened Beverages

Now that you know how many sugar-sweetened drinks, water, and dairy products your children consume in a day, you are ready to begin weaning them off of sugar-sweetened beverages, one kind at a time. The reason for identifying what they currently drink is to make sure that when you remove one type of drink—juice, for example—they don't start drinking more soda to replace the sugar they are missing.

At the end of the chapter we have provided instructions for creating calen-dars for each type of beverage they consume. You can write the beginning amounts followed by how much they will drink each day until they reach their goal on these calendars. They can serve as motivating tools if you hang them where your children can see them. These tools will help them stick to the program as well.

3. Follow Their Lead

We have prescribed an order for eliminating or reducing the types of beverages your child drinks. We recommend that order, but if it doesn't feel right or if you sense that you should tackle soda before juice, for example, feel free to do so. If it will help your teen or tween to follow the program you may want to ask him to choose which drinks he wants to limit first. The order is not essential as long as at the end of this step you have limited juice, eliminated all other sugar-sweetened beverages, switched to plain milk, and added water to your child's diet.

4. Give Them Enough Time

The time it takes for children to reach the goal will vary depending on how many beverages and the type of beverages they drink every day. Young children who do not drink caffeinated beverages will most likely finish within a month, but older children who consume a lot of sugar-laden drinks that contain caffeine may take longer because they need to be weaned off of their caffeine intake slowly in order to reduce the intensity of potential withdrawal symptoms.

On average, it will take three to four weeks to accomplish reaching the goal for juice, flavored milk, sports drinks, and flavored water. If your children drink a huge amount or refuse to switch from flavored milk to plain, it is fine if it takes longer to reach the goal as long as you decrease the amount of sweetened beverages each day by the required amount. When eliminating caffeinated drinks (cola, energy drinks, coffee, and tea), decreasing by only one drink per week is advised to lessen the side effects of stopping caffeine. If your teen consumes four caffeinated beverages a week it may take one month just to get off of these beverages alone.

Prescription for Limiting Juice

If your child drinks more than ½ cup (120 ml) of 100 percent juice a day (six years old and younger) or 1 cup (235 ml) of 100 percent juice (seven years old and older) or drinks juice with added sugar, then he or she needs to follow this step. If your child drinks the recommended amount or less of 100 percent juice, go to the next part: limiting flavored milk.

1 Switch to 100 Percent Juice

Switch to 100 percent juice products if your children drink juice cocktail, juice beverages, juice punch, juice-ades, and juice drinks. Serve your children products that only say "100 percent juice" on the label. Once your children are accustomed to the new 100 percent juice, you are ready to begin lowering the amount of juice they drink. Most children do not have a hard time or even notice a switch to 100 percent juice unless they have a favorite in which there are no 100 percent juice alternatives (Hawaiian Punch, for example).

They may give you a hard time when you switch to 100 percent juice, but be strong and consistent, providing a reward for added encouragement. Let them know they may have 100 percent juice or no juice at all. They may refuse to drink the new juice: in this case, you will have automatically completed this section and can move on to reducing flavored milk. Just make sure they eat two servings of fruit a day.

2 Dilute Juice to Tolerance (Optional)

It is easier on children when weaning them off of too much juice to dilute their juice first. This way, they do not notice a change and you can subtly adjust their taste buds to become accustomed to and like the less-sweet taste of diluted juice.

Diluting your children's juice is possible if you serve them juice from a large container at home or pour their juice for them into a glass. You will need a measuring cup that measures in ounces to dilute their juice for this step. It won't be possible to dilute if your child drinks juice from a juice box or other single-serving container. It is best if you can get your child accustomed to the taste of diluted juice over time but if not, jump to Step 3: Reduce the Amount of Juice. Following, you will learn how to dilute their juice.

In a glass or cup: Replace 1 ounce (28 ml) of juice with 1 ounce (28 ml) of water in every 8-ounce (235 ml) cup of juice that your children drink without telling them. If they know that you are diluting their juice, they will not want to try it. If you can keep it from them, at least for the first couple of dilutions, then before they know it they will get used to a less sugary taste and a non-syruplike consistency. For older children, add water to the large jug of juice slowly and once they get used to it, you can tell them what you have done. For fun, do a side-by-side comparison of the old versus new diluted juice so they can see and taste the difference. Continue to dilute their juice by replacing 1 ounce of juice with 1 ounce of water each day thereafter until they notice. Once they notice you can tell them what you have been doing and why, then go back up to the last dilution that they liked.

In a large juice container: Add ½ cup (120 ml) of water to a quart (liter) of juice on day one. Add another ½ cup (120 ml) of water every day thereafter until your child complains. Once she does, back up a step by adding ½ cup (120 ml) less water until she finds the juice palatable again. This concentration of juice is what you will use in the next step of reducing the amount.

3 Reduce the Amount of Juice

You don't need to dilute your children's juice before moving on to this step, but it is worth a try. Here's how to reduce their juice intake:

Reduce the total amount of pure juice that your children drinks by ¼ cup (2 ounces [60 ml]) a day for children six years and younger and ½ cup (4 ounces [120 ml]) per day for children seven years of age and older. You can take two or three days between reductions if your child has a huge issue with this step.

Once your children reach the following daily juice consumption totals, they will have reached their first goal: **½ cup (120 ml) of 100 percent fruit juice for children six and younger** and **1 cup (235 ml) of 100 percent fruit juice for children seven and older**.

▶ **Note:** *Your children may be drinking 2 cups (475 ml) of juice a day in total if it is diluted. The goal listed previously is the amount of undiluted juice they can have—how much you dilute it is up to you and them.*

4 Reduce the Number of Juice Boxes

If your children drink mostly juice boxes, first switch to 100 percent juice box juice. Once they are used to the taste, reduce the number of boxes they drink by one every three days until you reach one juice box a day. Make sure that you are serving age-appropriate juice box sizes because they range from a little more than 4 ounces (120 ml) which are great for kids under four to 6¾ ounces (190 ml) for the older child. The juice box counts toward their daily limit of **½ cup (120 ml) of 100 percent fruit juice for children six and younger** and **1 cup (235 ml) of 100 percent fruit juice for children seven and older**.

✔ Summary

☐ Switch to 100 percent juice.

☐ (Optional) Dilute 100 percent juice with 1 ounce (28 ml) of water every day until tolerance.

☐ Reduce juice intake every one to three days by 2 ounces (60 ml) for children six and younger and by 4 ounces for children seven and older until the goal of 4 ounces (120 ml) per day (six years and younger) or 8 ounces (235 ml) per day (seven years and older) is met.

☐ Reduce the number of juice boxes until the goal is met.

Children who drink flavored milk or flavored milk alternatives should follow this step. Children who drink just plain milk or no milk at all can skip this step and go on to eliminating soda and energy drinks.

The goal is to eliminate flavored milk from your children's diet. After they have finished the program, you may use it as a sweet treat once in a while, but your mission now is to get them used to the taste of plain milk. Flavored milk includes chocolate-, vanilla-, and strawberry-flavored cow's milk and chocolate, carob, and some vanilla varieties of soy, rice, almond, or coconut milk. Reduce their intake of flavored milk and replace it with low-fat or nonfat plain milk two or three times a day (whole milk for children one to two years of age) as long as your child tolerates milk well. The following are recommended amounts of milk that a child should consume daily if you rely on dairy products to provide calcium in your child's diet:

- 2 to 3 years old: 2 cups (475 ml) plain milk a day
- 4 to 8 years old: 2½ cups (600 ml) plain milk a day
- 9 to 13 years old: 3 cups (700 ml) plain milk day
- 14 to 18 years old: 3 cups (700 ml) plain milk day

1 Stop Flavored Milk Outside the Home

Start by determining the amount of flavored milk that your children drink in a day and where they get their milk from. If your children get flavored milk at school, start by having them switch to plain milk at school. Some schools have electronic purchasing systems in place that prohibit children from purchasing certain items that parents select, but the majority of schools do not. You will have to rely on the honor system (with rewards) if your school has no procedure in place to stop your child from getting flavored milk. The purpose of this step is to get ready to dilute their flavored milk at home because it is confusing for children to drink one type of milk in one setting and another at home.

Reduce chocolate and other flavored milk outside the home by 1 cup (235 ml) or one 6- to 8-ounce (175 to 235 ml) box every four days. Be sure to replace the flavored dairy that they were consuming outside the home with unflavored dairy products.

Once you have eliminated flavored milk that is consumed outside the home, go on to the next step: dilution.

2 Dilute Flavored Milk at Home (Optional)

As in the juice step, parents will need measuring cups that measure ounces. Dilute every glass of flavored milk that your child consumes.

By the glass or cup: Add 2 ounces (60 ml) of plain milk to 6 ounces (175 ml) of chocolate milk and see how your children react. If they can tolerate the less sweet taste, wait another two days for them to get used to the new taste and then dilute their milk by another ounce—add 3 ounces (90 ml) of plain milk to 5 ounces (150 ml) of flavored milk. Repeat diluting by 1 more ounce (28 ml) every two days until they have reached the goal and are drinking only plain milk or they have reached a point where they don't like the diluted

flavored drink anymore. If this is the case, back up a step and offer them the dilution they drank the day before.

You are now ready for the next step, reduction, using a dilution of flavored milk that they can tolerate. As with juice, it is not essential that your children drink diluted flavored milk before starting the next step. Diluting, in our experience, just makes it easier for a child to wean off of flavored milk. Your goal is to not only to remove chocolate milk (and other flavored milk) from your children's diet but also to replace flavored milk with plain milk because it is important that they continue to drink milk.

3 Reduce and Replace Flavored Milk

If your children currently drink plain milk and flavored milk: Reduce the total amount of flavored milk they drink (diluted or undiluted) each day by 1 ounce (⅛ cup [28 ml]) for younger children and 2 ounces (¼ cup [60 ml]) for older children at each serving until your children no longer drink any flavored milk. Continue to offer them plain milk during this step instead and make sure that each day they drink 2 to 3 cups (475 to 700 ml) of milk. At the end of this step, they will be drinking 2 to 3 cups (475 to 700 ml) of just plain milk.

If they drink only flavored milk: Reduce the total amount of flavored milk your children drink (diluted or undiluted) by 1 ounce (28 ml) for younger children and 2 ounces (60 ml) for older children at each serving. Substitute plain milk for the flavored milk you took away. For example, offer your child 2 ounces (60 ml) of plain milk in a glass for the 2 ounces (60 ml) of flavored milk you took away on the first day, and repeat for three more days until all you are offering is plain milk and no flavored milk. A good tool to encourage them to transition from flavored to unflavored milk is to use the flavored milk as an incentive: once they drink their 2 ounces (60 ml) of plain milk for lunch on day 1 they can drink their 6 ounces (175 ml) of flavored milk afterward. You can do the same at snack and dinner.

✔ Summary

☐ Outside the home: Reduce chocolate and other flavored milk boxes by one every four days until zero is reached.

☐ (Optional) Dilute flavored milk at home by 2 ounces (60 ml) of plain milk day and 1 ounce (28 ml) until your children react to the difference.

☐ Reduce 1 ounce (28 ml) of flavored milk (younger children) or 2 ounces (60 ml) of flavored milk (older children) a day and replace with plain milk until the goal is met, which is no flavored milk and 2 to 3 cups (475 to 700 ml) of plain milk a day.

Prescription for Eliminating Soda and Energy Drinks

Children should follow this step if they drink soda or energy drinks, including diet (sweetened with artificial sweeteners), regular, caffeinated, or decaffeinated drinks. If your child does not drink soda or energy drinks, go to the next program— sports drinks and flavored water.

1 Prepare the House

Have just enough soda or energy drinks in the house to wean your children off of them. Once they reach their goal of consuming no soda or energy drinks, stop buying them for the house because this will help reduce the temptation to drink them when your children are at home. Once you have broken your children's sugar addiction, you can reintroduce an occasional soda, but energy drinks should always be discouraged. These have been responsible for many health problems and emergency room visits, and you can view them as you would an alcoholic drink and forbid your child from drinking them until they are adults. For more on the health effects of these drinks, see the next section.

You may also want to consider reducing the amount of time your children watch television, or at least have them mute the television when advertisements come on. This is one way to decrease the influence that advertisers for these products have on your child. If your child is old enough, you might discuss other ways in which advertisers try to reach kids his age, such as with Internet pop-up ads, billboards at sports games, school sponsorships in exchange for computer equipment, and so on. Raising their awareness may help them better resist marketing efforts targeted toward their age group.

2 Reduce and Eliminate Noncaffeinated Beverages

Once you and your children are prepared, reduce decaffeinated soda consumption by one can or one 8-ounce (235 ml) glass every four days until they aren't drinking it anymore.

For older children especially, bribes may be necessary and very helpful in accomplishing this step. Kids like to be rewarded for their efforts just like adults do. For each can of soda or energy drink they stop drinking, offer them a reward or points that they can cash in at the end of the program for a big prize. We have included prize points on each handout to help you and your children keep track of their progress and motivate them to continue reducing sugar in their diet. Refer to chapter 1 for examples of age-appropriate prizes.

3 Reduce and Eliminate Caffeinated Soda and Energy Drinks

If your children consume caffeinated soda and energy drinks, reduce their intake by one drink (one can or 8 ounces [235 ml]) per week. If you are not sure whether your child's soda has caffeine, check the ingredient list. Give them one week before reducing their intake again. They need to take it slow to minimize caffeine withdrawal symptoms.

✔ Summary

☐ Prepare the house by removing or consuming the soda you keep on hand.

☐ Reduce decaffeinated soda consumption by one can or one 8-ounce (235 ml) glass every four days until they aren't drinking it anymore.

☐ Reduce caffeinated soda and all energy drinks by one can or one 8-ounce (235 ml) glass every seven days until they've reached the goal, which is no soda and no energy drinks.

Prescription for Eliminating Sports Drinks and Flavored Water

Your children should follow this step if they drink sports drinks or flavored water for casual consumption or after a regular workout, practice, or game. Consuming a sports drink after prolonged bouts of strenuous exercise or high heat and humidity that causes excess sweating is fine as long as it is necessary. If your child doesn't drink any sports drinks or flavored water, go to the next section: tea and coffee.

1 Bring Water to Sports Events

Begin by providing only plain water at sports events unless your child's pediatrician has recommended a sports drink. If sports drinks and flavored water are not available to them at games and when they are working out, your child will drink them less often. Make sure your child does not drink more of one drink (flavored water) when reducing another (sports drinks).

Have your child bring water with her to each sporting event. You can purchase a metal (preferred) or plastic water bottle to reuse over time. When purchasing plastic water bottles, make sure you look for brands that are BPA-free and have the number 2, 4, or 5 on the bottom of the container. Let your child pick an especially cool-looking one.

2 Reduce and Replace Sports Drinks

If your children drink sports drinks to quench their thirst during the day, reduce their sports drink consumption by ½ cup (120 ml) a day until they reach zero. Replace your children's sports drinks with plain water. For every ½ cup (120 ml) reduction, add ½ cup (120 ml) of water to their daily routine.

3 Replace Flavored Water with Plain Water

Replace flavored water with plain water by ½ cup (120 ml) a day until the goal of no flavored water is met. If your children will not drink plain water, add a slice of citrus or mint leaf to their water glass. Sometimes adding ice to water entices children to drink plain water. Always keep water easily accessible to encourage your children to drink it throughout the day. Put a pitcher of water with ice on the counter or leave it on the top shelf of the refrigerator to encourage them to drink it.

▶ **Note:** *Make sure your children maintain their goal between categories; once they eliminate soda and move on to sports drinks, for example, do not allow them to drink soda again. Feel free to take up to a week in between categories before making another change if your children are still adjusting to the current step.*

✔ Summary

☐ Bring plain water to sports events.

☐ Reduce sports drinks by ½ cup (120 ml) every day and replace with ½ cup (120 ml) of plain water until the goal is met (no sports drinks, unless prescribed by a pediatrician).

☐ Replace flavored water with plain water by ½ cup (120 ml) a day until the goal of no sweetened flavored water is met.

How Much Water Should Your Children Drink Each Day?

Make sure that your child gets at a minimum the following amount of plain water (or naturally flavored water that you make at home) every day:

Recommended Daily Water Intake for Kids

Age	Adequate daily beverage intake*	Minimum water requirement**
Children 2 to 3	4 cups (1 L)	1½ cups (355 ml) water (2 cups [475 ml] milk, ½ cup [120 ml] juice)
Children 4 to 6	5 cups (1.25 L)	2 cups (475 ml) water (2½ cups [590 ml] milk, ½ cup [120 ml] juice)
Children 7 to 8	5 cups (1.25 L)	1½ cups (355 ml) water (2½ cups [600 ml] milk, 1 cup [235 ml] juice)
Boys 9 to 13	8 cups (2 L)	4 cups (950 ml) water (3 cups [710 ml] milk, 1 cup [235 ml] juice)
Girls 9 to 13	7 cups (1.75 L)	3 cups (710 ml) water (3 cups [710 ml] milk, 1 cup [235 ml] juice)
Boys 14 to 18	11 cups (2.5 L)	7 cups (1.6 L) water (3 cups [710 ml] milk, 1 cup [235 ml] juice)
Girls 14 to 18	8 cups (2 L)	4 cups (950 ml) water (3 cups [710 ml] milk, 1 cup [235 ml] juice)

Source: *Dietary Reference Intakes: The Essential Guide to Nutrient Requirements, Water.* (Washington, DC: The National Academies Press, 2006), pp. 156–166. These are estimated requirements. If your children are thirsty, give them more. If they are playing in hot or humid weather, have a fever, are taking certain medications, or are exercising, their water requirement will increase.

*Adequate intake is based on median total water intake from U.S. survey data. Total beverage intake includes water plus the water your child will get from other beverages, such as milk and juice.

**Minimum water requirement is calculated by taking the adequate daily beverage intake listed to the left and subtracting from it the amount of juice and milk your child should drink every day (2 to 3 glasses of milk and ½ to 1 cup (120 to 235 ml) of juice). If your children drink more or less than the recommended amount of juice or dairy, adjust their water intake accordingly.

Your children should follow this step if they drink coffee, sugar-sweetened iced tea, and hot tea. If they don't drink any tea, iced tea, or coffee and have reached their goal for all sugar-sweetened beverages, they are ready to go to the next section on revamping breakfast.

1 Eliminate Hot and Iced Tea

Each week, replace 1 cup (235 ml) of hot or cold caffeinated tea with water. Continue to eliminate 1 cup (235 ml) of hot or cold caffeinated tea a week until zero is reached. It is okay to allow your child to drink one decaffeinated cup of tea a day as long as it is low in sugar. Children need to get most of their liquids from water and milk (if tolerated). Herbal or fruit teas with minimal added sugar are also fine—just make sure the herbal tea you choose is safe for children. For example, a child with ragweed allergies should stay away from chamomile tea.

Do not add any sweeteners to the tea, except for stevia or, at most, one teaspoon (4 g) of honey in 8 ounces (235 ml).

2 Eliminate Coffee

Reduce coffee drinks by one a week until zero is reached. Refer to the section on managing withdrawal symptoms, such as headaches and moodiness, when reducing caffeine intake. Make sure your children drink enough water during this step because it will help them manage side effects better if they are well hydrated.

✔ Summary

☐ Reduce hot and iced caffeinated tea by 1 cup (235 ml) a week until zero is reached.

☐ Reduce coffee drinks by one a week until zero is reached.

Healthy Drink Options for Your Children

We both agree that water is the best drink for people. Dr. Deb does not encourage drinking products made with natural noncalorie sweeteners, whereas Dr. T feels this can be okay (see the next section for more on this topic). Dr. Deb's healthy beverage options include mixing your child's daily juice allotment with sparkling water or adding fruit slices or mint leaves to plain water to give it a subtle taste.

Dr. T encourages people to find a way to enjoy their vices healthfully and considers stevia to be a good solution. Some stevia products have natural flavors that allow a reasonable alternative to soda. For stevia, though, brand is critical, because poorly filtered brands taste, well, gross. There are a few well-made products that taste great. An excellent, readily available brand is SweetLeaf, and it can be found in most health food stores, more and more restaurants, and even some supermarkets. Zevia has a large selection of stevia-flavored sodas and is available in most health-food stores.

What You Can Do When Your Children Go through Sugar and Caffeine Withdrawal

Expect your children to go through a period of withdrawal from the lack of sugar and also, potentially, from caffeine if they consume enough to create a physical dependency. This program is designed to ease your children off of added sugar and caffeine to lessen the severity of their withdrawal symptoms. If they are having a hard time with withdrawal symptoms, you can always slow down the program and give them more time between steps to adjust and recuperate.

Children who are addicted to sugar can experience similar withdrawal symptoms as adults who are addicted to alcohol. There seems to be many similarities between sugar and alcohol addiction, and research is continuing to uncover links between the two. Children with an alcoholic parent, especially an alcoholic father, are more susceptible to developing a strong preference for sweet tastes. Sugar withdrawal symptoms may include, but are not limited to, the following.

- Moodiness
- Anxiety
- Anger outbursts
- Weepiness
- Headaches
- Shakiness
- Intense hunger and/or cravings

To minimize these withdrawal symptoms, try the following.

Provide a well-balanced diet. Make sure your children eat a well-balanced diet with sufficient protein to reduce withdrawal symptoms. If you find your children are shaky, moody, weepy, or just not themselves, offer them a healthy snack with whole grains or vegetables and protein (refer to chapter 4 for great snack ideas). The nutrients that these foods supply will help regulate their blood sugar level over the long run.

Give them space. The best thing you can do is give your children the space they need to act out their frustration and moodiness. Meet anger, frustration, and downright crankiness with patience and kindness. This will be easier to do if you are well rested and prepared.

Provide lots of water. Being well hydrated will help your children feel better. Try giving your children soothing tea, such as chamomile (German chamomile), unless they have a ragweed allergy, to help them calm down and center during this time. You can even serve it cold to drink throughout the day.

Have them take a multivitamin/mineral supplement. We also recommend children take a multivitamin/mineral supplement every day to ensure they are getting the micronutrients they need. When buying a vitamin for your child, make sure it is age-appropriate and designed for children. Aim for 100 percent to 150 percent of the daily value (% DV) of each nutrient, unless otherwise recommended by a health practitioner.

Make sure they get enough sleep. Children will need extra sleep during periods of withdrawal. Encourage them to get to bed early and nap if possible. The following are daily sleep requirements:

2 to 3 years old: 12 to 14 hours
4 to 5 years old: 11 to 13 hours
6 to 12 years old: 10 to 11 hours
Adolescents: 8½ to 9¼ hours

Get them to exercise and go outside. Make sure your children exercise for at least an hour a day. They need to burn off and settle their energy, plus the endorphins that are released during exercise will help them feel better after they finish. The fresh air and sunshine will also help lift their mood.

Part II
The Lowdown on Liquid Sugar

What you should know, but probably don't, about the health hazards of liquid sugar

Children need to drink fluids every day to keep hydrated, but certain drinks can potentially be toxic, even at low levels. The soda and energy drinks they often consume provide few nutrients and often contain massive amounts of sugar, phosphoric acid, and caffeine, which can be dangerous for children.

Other beverages are not toxic, but should be consumed in moderation because too much can lead to excess caloric intake and complications like weight gain and the development of diabetes. Juice, for example, can be part of a healthy diet as long as you limit and water down the amount that your child drinks in a day. Plain milk is a great source of calcium and protein, but flavored milk delivers too much sugar. We have written this section to help you make sense of the beverage choices out there—which drinks your children can consume daily, which ones they should limit, and which ones they should avoid altogether.

What Kids Should Drink Every Day

Water is an essential component of your child's diet and is needed for almost every bodily function. Approximately 60 to 70 percent of your child's body weight is made up of water.

Children need to replace the water they lose daily from sweating, breathing, pooping, and urinating. Do not rely on thirst as a good early indicator of dehydration. By the time children say they are thirsty they may already be dehydrated. Instead, make sure they have healthy drinks available to them throughout the day that they can easily get to. Perhaps some of the moodiness and fatigue in your child or teen stems from dehydration. We have seen many children go from being cranky couch potatoes to pleasant, energetic beings when they become hydrated.

The chart on the following page shows the beverage amounts that your child should consume in a day. If your child exercises, has a chronic illness, is on certain medications, or is exposed to hot weather, he or she will need more water than what is recommended in the chart.

A good rule of thumb is to explain to children that when they have enough water, their urine is light yellow or clear. Bright yellow, strong-smelling urine may be a sign of dehydration. (Exceptions include if they take a vitamin B complex, which makes urine bright yellow, and eating asparagus, which gives urine an odor.)

Recommended Daily Liquid Intake for Healthy Children

Beverage	Age					
	Children 2 to 3	Children 4 to 8	Boys 9 to 13	Girls 9 to 13	Boys 14 to 18	Girls 14 to 18
Water	1½ cups (355 ml)	2 cups (475 ml) (4 to 6 years) / 1½ cups (355 ml) (7 to 8 years)	4 cups (950 ml)	3 cups (710 ml)	7 cups (1.6 L)	4 cups (950 ml)
Milk*	2 cups (475 ml)	2½ cups (600 ml)	3 cups (710 ml)	3 cups (710 ml)	3 cups (710 ml)	3 cups (710 ml)
Juice	½ cup (120 ml)	½ cup (120 ml) (4 to 6 years) / 1 cup (235 ml) (7 to 8 years)	1 cup (235 ml)	1 cup (235 ml)	1 cup (235 ml)	1 cup (235 ml)
Daily total	4 cups (0.9 L)	5 cups (1.2 L)	8 cups (1.8 L)	7 cups (1.6 L)	11 cups (2.6 L)	8 cups (1.8 L)

Source: U.S. Department of Agriculture and Institute of Medicine DRI for Water by Life Group
*Low-fat or 1 percent milk for children two years and older

The Reality of Artificial Sweeteners

In an attempt to lower the amount of added sugar in beverages, manufacturers have added artificial sweeteners to many drinks on the market. These artificial sweeteners include the following.

- Acesulfame potassium (acesulfame K, Sunnett, Sweet One)
- Aspartame (NutraSweet, Equal)
- Sucralose (Splenda)
- Saccharine (Sweet'N Low, Necta Sweet)
- Neotame

Beat Sugar Addiction Now for Kids

Look at the ingredient list to determine whether a product contains artificial sweeteners. It most likely does if you see any of the following words on the label: "lite," "light," "0 calorie," and "Zero." We do not recommend giving children beverages with artificial sweeteners for the following reasons:

- Even though artificial sweeteners are generally recognized as safe by the U.S. Food and Drug Administration, they have not been extensively studied in children over time. In fact, long-term studies on the consumption of artificial sweeteners by adults are also lacking, and they may be quite toxic.
- Children's brains are still developing after birth and as such are sensitive to chemicals that adults may not have an issue with.
- Artificial sweeteners set up your child's taste buds to crave sweeter tasting items and develop a taste for foods and beverages with artificially high sweet tastes. Kids need to get used to the natural, subtler, sweet taste of fruits and vegetables to train their taste buds to eat and prefer healthy food and drinks.

NATURALLY LOW SUGAR AND SUGAR-FREE SWEETENERS

Whether or not you should let your child consume natural, sugar-free sweeteners during this program is a point that the authors disagree on. Dr. T feels that it is important for children to have things they can enjoy and recognizes that everything has its own pros and cons. Dr. Deb thinks that the use of these sweeteners trains kids' palates to crave more sweet-tasting foods and thus prefer these foods to naturally sweet fruit and vegetables.

Dr. T says: Although water is the healthiest drink, kids are kids and I think it's good for them to have healthy alternatives (adults as well). I consider both stevia and erythritol to be healthy, including Truvia and PureVia. SweetLeaf stevia tastes the best (other brands are bitter) and is pure stevia. As with most things, consuming these sweeteners is a matter of balance and degree.

There are sodas that are natural and sweetened with stevia. These are quite sweet and the colas are acidic, so I would limit children to one (or perhaps two) a day. These stevia-sweetened sodas are made by Zevia (see Zevia.com), and I suspect other companies will be entering the market. These are available at most health food stores.

In addition, I feel it is okay to make lemonade sweetened with stevia to keep in your refrigerator. The brand of stevia is critical because if it is not filtered, it will taste bitter. I recommend either a liquid stevia from Body Ecology (800-4-stevia) or SweetLeaf stevia (available at most health food stores). You can combine 3 to 4 cups (700 to 950 ml) of water, ¼ cup (60 ml) of lemon juice, and stevia to taste. Making caffeine-free iced tea from tea bags and adding stevia is also a tasty, healthy, and refreshing drink.

Although fruit juices have the same ¾ teaspoon of sugar per ounce (28 ml) as regular sodas do, 4 to 8 ounces (120 to 235 ml) a day is okay. If you water it down and add a little stevia, 8 ounces (235 ml) of juice can become 80 ounces (2.5 L) of a healthy drink. To put this in perspective, products labeled "fruit drinks" usually are only 10 percent juice and 90 percent added water. The trick? Water the juice down slowly over time, so your child's taste buds can adapt.

Although I agree with Dr. Deb that it's important for the taste buds to adapt to a normal, natural sweetness level, I also recognize the reality that children live where they are not under our watchful eyes. My preference is to give them choices, including ones that combine pleasure and health.

Dr. Deb says: There are some sugar substitutes that are natural and contain little to no calories. Stevia, erythritol, and a combination of the two, Truvia and PureVia, are examples. Because one of the major goals of eliminating sugary beverages from your children's diet is to retrain their taste buds to prefer less sugary food and drink, consuming a lot of these sugar substitutes is not a good idea, at least during the program.

Think of the analogy of your children sledding: once they start down the hill, it is hard to stop. Once you start to sneak in sweet-tasting food and drinks, you push your children's preference for sweetness close to, if not over, the edge of them wanting and craving sweet items. Natural sweeteners have a sweet taste that differs from that found in fruits and vegetables and sets our kids' taste buds to want overly sweet tastes. Stevia can be 300 times sweeter than sugar.

I also am cautious when substances we add to food act differently in our bodies than foods we have been eating for eons. Erythritol is a sugar alcohol and is absorbed from the small intestine and excreted unchanged mostly through the urine. This seems like a lot of needless work for the kidneys with no added benefit for the body. Food is, by nature, designed to be absorbed from the gut and the nutrients used by the cells in the body. The brain is also designed to respond to an increase or decrease in the amount of calories we take in based on the intricate feedback loop between the food we eat, the sugar levels that follow, and the messages that are sent to the brain. We do not yet know enough about the long-term consequences of consuming artificial sweeteners on this feedback mechanism in our children's brains.

In summary, I don't think we know enough about the long-term consequences of natural noncalorie sweeteners to recommend them regularly for healthy children, but they do serve a purpose for children with diabetes.

In raising kids, it is common for the parents to have different perspectives, just as it is in medicine. Either of the preceding choices is okay. We both recommend finding the approach that works best for you and your children.

Do Kids Need Juice?

Children do not need to drink juice as long as they eat enough whole fruits each day (see the chart in this chapter for the daily recommended serving amount of fruit servings for children). Juice provides no additional nutritional benefits over eating whole fruit and because excess consumption can lead to the intake of too many sugar calories, short stature, and unexplained abdominal pain, moderation is important. The USDA's *Dietary Guidelines for Americans, 2010* states that *the majority of the fruit that is recommended should come from whole fruit, not juice.*

Juice lacks the fiber that fruit contains, so it's easy to overindulge. Did you ever see a child eat two or three apples at one sitting? Probably not, but you have most likely observed children drink three or four juice boxes at a time, especially during birthday parties. The fiber in the fruit tells the child's belly that it is full, giving a signal to the brain that he or she has had enough. Juice bypasses this signal, so it is much easier to overdo the amount of juice that a child drinks than it is to overeat whole fruit.

Juice in its pure form is made up of mostly water followed by sugar (fructose, glucose, sucrose, and sorbitol), and a modest amount of certain vitamins and minerals. Your child would have to eat as many as eight oranges to get the amount of sugar in a 16-ounce (450 ml), no-sugar-added glass of orange juice! Because juice is high in sugar and a favorite among children, the American Academy of Pediatrics (AAP) in 2007 decided to limit the amount of juice it recommends children drink: 4 to 6 ounces (120 to 175 ml) for children one to six years, and 8 to 12 ounces (235 to 355 ml) for children seven to eighteen years of age. The AAP does not recommend juice for babies under six months of age and for older babies only when they can drink it out of a cup. The academy does not advise drinking juice from a bottle. The following table lists daily fruit requirements.

How Much Fruit Should Children Eat Daily?

Age	USDA daily recommended amount
Children 2 to 3	1 cup (225 g)
Children 4 to 8	1 to 1½ cups (225 to 350 g)
Children 9 to 13	1½ cups (350 g)
Boys 14 to 18	2 cups (450 g)
Girls 14 to 18	1½ cups (350 g)

Source: U.S. Department of Agriculture

WHAT TYPE OF JUICE SHOULD MY CHILD DRINK?

- Stick with 100 percent juice. Do not be fooled by labels that say "made with juice" or "contains juice."
- Avoid juice cocktails, juice drinks, juice punch, and juice beverages because they can contain as little as 10 percent real juice with sugar or juice concentrate added.
- Avoid juice that is sold as "50 percent less sugar" and "light" because they usually have artificial sweeteners added to it. Make light juice yourself by diluting 100 percent juice with water.
- Avoid fruit smoothies because these can pack 31 grams of sugar per cup.
- Be careful of juice that is made from concentrate because it can pack more sugar in each serving of juice unless it says "water sufficient to reconstitute." What this means is that the manufacturer added enough water back to the concentrate to create the same proportion of water to sugar as found in 100 percent juice.

What to Do When Your Child Wants a Liquid Meal

Many children, especially younger children, prefer to drink their calories instead of eating them. They show up at the dinner table and down several glasses of their favorite beverage and have little to no room for dinner. If this sounds like your child, you will want to separate drinking from eating by offering milk between meals.

Make sure your children drink enough throughout the day so they are well hydrated when they show up for meals. Offer them milk and water at snack time and make sure that snack time is at least 2 hours before mealtime so that they don't fill up on beverages and have no room for the meal. At the table, pour a small glass of water (½ cup [120 ml] for younger children and 1 cup [235 ml] for older) for them to drink during the meal. Once they have finished eating their food, offer them a glass of milk. If they are full after their meal, serve them milk the next time they are hungry.

Using the beverage that they prefer as a motivator to eat their meal works for children who prefer to drink their calories. Even young children get the concept of "first this then that": First eat your meal, and then you can have your milk. Do not offer juice, soda, or other sweetened beverages at mealtime, with the exception being juice at breakfast. These are just empty calories that fill up your child who instead needs to eat nutrient-rich meals.

- Juice that is made from vegetable and fruit juice has less sugar than juice made from just pure fruit. It can be a healthy choice, but you still need to limit it to one serving a day and it does not count as a vegetable serving.
- Juice can say "unsweetened" on the label yet contain lots of added sugar in the form of juice concentrate. Be careful when selecting those varieties.
- Look for varieties of juice that have about 22 grams (5½ teaspoons) of sugar per 8 ounces (235 ml) of juice. That would equal 28 grams (7 teaspoons) of sugar per 10-ounce (285 ml) serving, 17 grams (4¼ teaspoons) of sugar per 6-ounce (175 ml) serving, 19 grams (4¾ teaspoons) of sugar per 6¾-ounce (200 ml) juice box, or 12 grams (3 teaspoons) of sugar per 4¼-ounce (125 ml) mini juice box.

The Skinny on Milk

Dairy products are the number one source of calcium in a child's diet. If children do not get enough calcium while they are growing and putting down the foundation that makes their bones strong, they risk developing weak bones for their entire life. In fact, children's bodies are uniquely designed before the age of twenty to absorb and deposit more calcium into their bones. By the time a boy reaches age twenty and a girl age eighteen, they have acquired almost 90 percent of their adult bone mass. Think of children's bones as little banks: they can make calcium deposits before age twenty but after that, mostly withdrawals.

As children age, they start to replace the milk they were used to drinking with soda and other sugar-sweetened beverages. Low calcium intake is found in children age nine and older and especially in adolescent girls. This group is particularly vulnerable to developing low bone mass, which can lead to osteoporosis later in life.

Consuming milk has also been found to decrease the risk of developing metabolic syndrome, which affects insulin resistance and glucose intolerance. In many studies, milk was also shown to reduce the risk of coronary artery disease and ischemic stroke. In terms of adverse effects, milk consumption is related to the development of prostate cancer in men, and the jury is still out but it may increase the risk of ovarian cancer in women.

Even though milk can be a healthy food in a child's diet (depending on which expert you ask), it is not essential. If your child has symptoms of milk allergies or intolerance, such as stomachaches or a lot of gas, or simply doesn't like it, consider this: humans are the only species that continues to drink milk after they are weaned, and many of us, as we age, lose the ability to digest the sugar (lactose) found in milk. This suggests that milk is an option but simply not essential, especially if your child gets sunshine to make vitamin D, exercises to increase bone density, and eats healthfully.

In addition, if your children have recurrent ear infections (and sometimes even if they have a constant runny nose with green mucus), there is a good chance that they have an allergy to milk protein, which can cause swelling and congestion in the nose and ears that results in recurrent infections. These children are then given antibiotics time and time again. Unfortunately, this repeated use of antibiotics can trigger candida/yeast overgrowth, which compounds the problem.

Sadly, standard medicine has a poor record of treating recurrent ear infections. Instead, try these steps:

1. Eliminate milk and cheese products from your child's diet for a month or two to see whether this helps. Be sure to give your child calcium-fortified soy or almond milk instead.
2. Cut back on sugar in your child's diet.

Very often, following these two steps will knock out the ear infections. If they do, you may need to limit your child's intake of milk products if the ear infections recur. If the problem persists after six weeks, see a holistic physician or NAET practitioner (www.naet.com) who can treat your child for milk allergies and candida.

One 8-ounce (235 ml) cup of plain milk contains 12 grams (3 teaspoons) of sugar in the form of lactose and has no added sugar. When flavors and sugar are added to plain milk, the sugar content rises to 20 to 30 grams (5 to 7½ teaspoons) per cup. This extra sugar adds up over time. If your child drinks just one glass of chocolate milk a day, that adds an extra 15 to 34 cups (3 to 7 kg) of sugar per year, depending on the brand. Double or triple that amount if your child has two or three glasses of chocolate milk a day. The same is true for vanilla- and strawberry-flavored milk. You wouldn't think that vanilla milk would contain a lot of added sugar, but it does, sometimes more so than strawberry milk.

GETTING THE CALCIUM WITHOUT THE SUGAR

Nutritionists and school personnel hotly debate whether the added sugar in flavored milk is a small price to pay to get kids to drink milk and thus get calcium. Many school districts are fighting over whether to remove flavored milk from their menus. We believe the extra sugar in flavored milk is too high a price to pay. There are other great sources of calcium besides milk, such as dark green leafy vegetables, white beans, and almonds. Also, numerous products nowadays are fortified with calcium, including tofu, some cereals, and soy milk.

If your child does not tolerate dairy and consumes any of the milk alternatives available on the market, like rice, soy, almond, or coconut milks, the same rules apply when these drinks are flavored. For some of these dairy alternatives, the vanilla-flavored drink has little added sugar while others have more than double the amount of added sugar than the plain varieties.

The following table will give you a sense of what to look for when choosing among the many varieties and brands of these milk alternatives. Look for brands that provide the lowest amount of sugar on the list: Make sure you select those with 10 grams (2½ teaspoons) or less per 8-ounce (235 ml) serving. Rice milk has the most sugar on this list, so you may want to switch to one of the other alternatives. If your child is accustomed to the taste of rice milk, you can make a low-sugar mixture by adding some soy, coconut, or almond milk to the rice milk until he gets used to the new taste.

The Amount of Sugar in Milk Alternatives

Milk alternative	Grams of sugar in 8 ounces (235 ml) of original/unflavored alternative	Grams of sugar in 8 ounces (235 ml) of vanilla-flavored alternative
Soy milk	4 to 7 g (1 to 1¾ teaspoons)	8 to 16 g (2 to 4 teaspoons)
Rice milk	10 to 14 g (2½ to 3½ teaspoons)	12 to 14 g (3 to 3½ teaspoons)
Almond milk	5 to 7 g (1 to 1¾ teaspoons)	9 to 15 g (2¼ to 3¾ teaspoons)
Coconut milk	6 g (1½ teaspoons)	7 to 9 g (1¾ to 2¼ teaspoons)

Source: Nutrition Facts label on beverages

Shop wisely and look for brands that provide limited added sugar. The vanilla flavor provides about the same or slightly more sugar as the original flavor. In some cases, there are even unsweetened and "lite" varieties of these alternatives. In addition, make sure they provide 20 to 30 percent of the daily value (DV) for calcium along with some vitamin D, which helps the body absorb calcium. Look for vitamin D^2 or D^3, which is the more potent form of vitamin D, in the ingredients list. Most dairy products are fortified with vitamin D and provide 30 percent DV for calcium.

What Type of Milk Should I Buy?

- If your child can tolerate dairy products, stick to plain low-fat and nonfat (skim) milk. (Note: Children between one and two years need the fat in whole milk, and children under one should not drink dairy products at all.)
- Avoid all chocolate-, strawberry-, and carob-flavored milks, such as dairy, rice, soy, coconut, and almond varieties.
- Choose the low-sugar varieties of vanilla- and original-flavored rice, almond, soy, and coconut milk.
- If your child can tolerate the unsweetened varieties of almond, coconut, or soy milk, those are best because they have 0 grams of sugar.
- Search for milk alternative brands that have "lite" varieties, because they contain much less sugar.
- Beware of flavored milk products that use artificial sweeteners like acesulfame potassium and avoid those as well.
- Be sure to buy dairy and milk alternative products that are fortified with vitamin D.

The Dangers of Soda and Energy Drinks

Children reach for soda today as they used to reach for a glass of water. In the past fifty years, soft drink consumption has increased 500 percent while serving sizes have more than tripled. These beverages are being marketed to children, who are easily influenced by the lure of the advertisements. Soda companies spend almost $500 million a year trying to influence your kids to buy sugar-sweetened drinks. Children get the message from these ads that it is cool to drink soda and energy drinks. They also watch their friends consuming soda and they want to follow suit. Besides the draw of the sweet taste of these drinks, many tweens and teens reach for the caffeinated soda and energy drinks for the buzz they get off of the caffeine, today's most popular stimulant.

Kids can choose from more than 400 types of soda, and they can buy these sugary drinks most places they go. Luckily, children in some public elementary and middle schools can no longer buy soda, but most teens still have access to diet soda and sports drinks at school. Good progress has been made in the public school system to date, but water is better than diet sodas. Well-hydrated children learn better because they are more alert and better able to concentrate. Diet soda does not make the cut as an optimal source of hydration.

Consider these reasons for removing soda and energy drinks from your child's diet:

1. **They contain too much sugar.** Each 12-ounce (355 ml) can of soda provides approximately 10 teaspoons (2.5 g) of sugar. With the average teenage boy drinking two 12-ounce (710 ml) cans a day and girls 1.4 cans (445 ml), that adds up to 152 cups (or thirteen and a half 5-pound bags [30 kg]) of sugar a year for teen boys and 106 cups (or nine and a quarter 5-pound bags [21 kg]) for teen girls.

2. **Consumption of these beverages can lead to weight gain and obesity.** For each 12-ounce (355 ml) can of soda you consume over an eighteen-month period, your risk of obesity rises a whopping 60 percent.

3. **They raise the risk of developing type 2 diabetes.** One in three Caucasian children and one in two Hispanic or African American children are expected to develop diabetes in their lifetime.

4. **They can have a negative effect on blood sugar levels.** The caffeine in soda aggravates the swings in blood sugar that occur when your children consume a diet high in sugar. This makes it even more difficult for children to control their intake of sugar because they are seeking the highs and trying to avoid the lows.

5. **Milk consumption decreases when soda consumption rises.** This transition from milk to soft drinks occurs between third and eighth grade for most children. Because milk products are the number one source of calcium in most children's diets, this decrease in consumption leads to an inadequate intake of calcium.

6. **Children may develop weak bones.** The phosphoric acid found in soda has a negative effect on bones. Several studies have demonstrated that drinking cola is associated with lower bone mineral density (softer bones) and more bone fractures.

7. **Consumption can increase the risk of cavities.** The added sugar plus the acidity of soda (phosphoric acid or citric acid) and energy drinks (citric acid) erode and rot the enamel on children's teeth, which leads to cavities.

8. **These beverages contain caffeine in toxic amounts.** Certain varieties of soda (including Coca-Cola, Mountain Dew, Mello Yellow, Sun Drop, Barq's Root Beer, and Sunkist Orange) and most energy drinks contain caffeine. Children with diabetes, seizures, cardiac abnormalities, or mood and behavior disorders are especially vulnerable to the effects of caffeine. Caffeine can

   - Increase blood pressure
   - Increase heart rate
   - Increase rate of speech so you talk fast
   - Trigger an irregular heartbeat
   - Lead to increased motor activity, or the jitters
   - Increase urination
   - Increase anxiety in those with an anxiety disorder
   - Affect the development of the brain, in certain doses
   - Affect the muscle of the heart while it is developing, in certain doses
   - Lead to addiction
   - Disrupt sleep, which can affect performance at school and during sports

What Happens When You Take Away the Caffeine?

Below are symptoms that can arise when you remove caffeine from your child's diet:

- Headache
- Fatigue
- Decreased energy
- Drowsiness
- Decreased alertness
- Difficulty concentrating
- Decreased desire to socialize
- Flulike symptoms
- Depressed mood
- Irritability
- Decreased contentedness
- Muscle pain or stiffness
- Nausea or vomiting

You can avoid most of these withdrawal symptoms by simply tapering caffeine intake over time instead of stopping it suddenly. We provide one week between reductions because this is adequate for most children and it's what the American Academy of Pediatrics recommends. Your child can also follow the same advice for limiting caffeine withdrawal symptoms as are listed for reducing sugar withdrawal symptoms:

- Get enough rest
- Exercise daily
- Go outside daily for air and sunshine
- Drink lots of water
- Try withdrawal tea
- Take as much solitary time as needed to regroup

9. **Caffeine can potentially have a negative effect on the developing nervous system.** Because of this concern, a recommended daily limit has been set at 2.5 milligrams of caffeine per kilogram of body weight. That would translate into 68 milligrams for a 60-pound (27 kg) third-grader or 142 milligrams for a 125-pound teenager (57 kg). These are the maximum levels that are recommended, but it is still best for children to avoid caffeine altogether.

ENERGY LOAN SHARK DRINKS

We call energy drinks "energy loan sharks" because they take more from you than they give. Stimulants in these energy drinks cause an initial increase in energy, but that energy spike is short lived. Long-term use can deplete the body of energy and make your child more tired. We have never seen energy drinks help a child become healthy and vibrant—rather, we often see jittery kids who have trouble handling the excess sugar and stimulants, which leads to trouble sleeping, moodiness, and other issues.

Energy drinks are a class of beverages unto themselves, and they are the most dangerous. Overdoses of energy drinks have been reported in children as young as five. Although the FDA limits the amount of caffeine found in soda, energy drinks are considered dietary supplements and as such there is no limit to the amount of caffeine they can contain. What is alarming is that 30 to 50 percent of adolescents and young adults report consuming energy drinks and more will soon, because energy drinks are the fastest growing market in the beverage industry in the United States.

Energy drinks contain carbohydrates in the form of added sugar (usually glucose or fructose forms) and stimulants, plus a combination of artificial flavors, added colors, benzoic and citric acid, electrolytes, vitamins, and other non-nutritive additives. The amount of added sugar varies widely in energy drinks, from sugar-free drinks with artificial sweeteners and no added sugar to others that provide a whopping 67 grams (16¾ teaspoons or about ⅓ cup) of sugar.

We have all been brainwashed to believe that getting more energy is as easy as picking up a beverage or food bar that is often loaded with sugar, nutrients, and stimulants. A quick energy fix is a misnomer because energy is created or sustained long-term by eating a healthy diet, exercising, getting adequate rest, and dealing with stressors in everyday life. A quick burst is only that—a jolt to the system and your child's body will become depleted if she stresses her body repeatedly by consuming these artificial drinks.

Stimulants in energy drinks often include caffeine, guarana, and ginseng. Guarana is a plant extract high in caffeine that we refer to as "herbal speed." It has three times the amount of caffeine as coffee and there have been reports that guarana can cause difficulty urinating, abdominal cramps, vomiting, spasms, and even heart arrhythmias. Some children are at high risk from the side effects of stimulants and you may or may not even know whether your child is susceptible until it is too late.

Other nonnutritive additives found in energy drinks that claim to increase energy and decrease fatigue include taurine, L-carnitine, creatine, and glucuro-nolactone. Taurine, an amino acid added to sports and energy drinks, has an effect on the heart similar to that of caffeine. As such, ingesting too much can be potentially harmful to your child. There is no benefit to children from ingesting excess taurine or other single amino acids in energy drinks because they get enough protein and amino acids from their diet. The amount of vitamins added are usually too low to be helpful.

Consuming energy drinks seems like a huge risk to take, and for what, a sweet-tasting beverage? There are plenty of healthier alternatives out there.

Young children should avoid caffeine altogether. The maximum daily levels are based on body weight: 45 milligrams of caffeine is the limit for a child who weighs 40 pounds (18 kg), 68 milligrams for a 60-pound child (27 kg), and 142 milligrams for a 125-pound (57 kg) teen. The following table lists the amounts of caffeine found in common beverages.

Beat Sugar Addiction Now for Kids

How Much Caffeine Are We Drinking?

Beverage	Serving size	Caffeine
Brewed coffee	8 oz (235 ml)	136 mg
Iced tea	8 oz (235 ml)	15 to 30 mg
Tea (green or black)	8 oz (235 ml)	48 mg
Decaf tea	8 oz (235 ml)	3 to 5 mg
Coca-Cola	12 oz (355 ml)	34 mg
Diet Coke	12 oz (355 ml)	46 mg
Pepsi	12 oz (355 ml)	39 mg
Mountain Dew	12 oz (355 ml)	55 mg
Jolt	12 oz (355 ml)	140 mg
Hot cocoa	8 oz (235 ml)	10 mg
Chocolate milk	8 oz (235 ml)	12 mg
Chocolate candy bar	1 bar (4.4 oz [123 g])	7 to 26 mg

Source: *Food and Chemical Toxicology*, 1996; *Journal of Food Science*, 2007; www. joltenergy.com, accessed January 2012.

Children vary in their ability to handle caffeine. Some children are very sensitive and the smallest amount of caffeine makes their heart beat faster and they become jittery; others can consume a lot with little effect. Children can develop a tolerance over time, as with other drugs, especially if they consume caffeine regularly. This means that children need more and more caffeine to feel the same effects as they did in the beginning because their body gets used to it. This can lead to your child consuming toxic amounts of caffeine. In fact, more than half of the calls regarding caffeine that the Poison Control Center received in 2005 concerned children.

Is There a Place for Sports Drinks and Flavored Water?

Sports drinks are meant to replenish the water and electrolytes that are lost from sweating during prolonged bouts of exercise plus add back some of the carbohydrates that are burned during activity. They are not meant for casual daily consumption. Most sports drinks contain carbohydrates in the form of added sugar, electrolytes, some minerals, and flavors. The electrolytes added most often include potassium and sodium, which most children get plenty of from their diet. Sports drinks almost always have artificial colors and flavors added to them, and if they have "Zero" on the label, they contain artificial sweeteners as well.

When adolescents were questioned on their use of sports and energy drinks, they said they used them both interchangeably and most did not distinguish between a sports drink designed to replenish electrolytes, water, and carbohydrates and an energy drink that contains stimulants. This suggests that children are reaching for energy drinks to hydrate and perform better during exercise when what they most often need is just water and, occasionally, a sports drink.

To begin reducing sports drinks, start by educating your child on the differences between a sports drink and an energy drink, along with the potential harmful effects of consuming energy drinks. Next, determine whether your child exercises hard and long enough to warrant needing a sports drink. You can use your own judgment or ask your child's pediatrician for guidance. Do your children exercise hard for more than an hour at a time? Do they sweat a

Once a product requires a laboratory to make the ingredients instead of Mother Nature, it has entered unhealthy territory.

lot because they play in hot and humid weather? If so, they may need a sports drink to replenish the electrolytes lost from sweating.

If your children do not seem to have the stamina to play well during sports or they do not seem to reach their potential and tire easily, the cause may be their diet. Eating a diet high in sugar will affect your child's performance during sports, and a sports drink will not fix the highs and lows in energy that children experience from a diet high in sugar. You can never replace a well-balanced diet with supplements or beverages that are marketed to enhance energy. It is like building a house on sand—it will fall down eventually. Make sure your child eats a well-balanced diet first, and then investigate the need to add sports drinks to their exercise routine later.

Why Flavored Water Isn't a Good Alternative

Most of us know that we need to drink water every day to stay healthy. The only problem is that some kids, especially if they have trained their taste buds to prefer sweet things, don't like the taste of water. It tastes bland or "yucky." We end up fighting with them day in and day out to drink their water. We add some to juice to their water and hope the water they get from fruits and veggies will be enough. Then we discover flavored water and away goes the fighting and pleading. Our children can drink flavored water without coaxing and, as a bonus, the water even has vitamins added to it. How can that be unhealthy?

If it sounds too good to be true, trust us, it almost always is, especially in the world of food. The best foods and drinks for our family have been around for thousands of years, but it seems as if we keep waiting for something new: a product that will taste so good that we don't have to fight our children to get them to eat or drink it. Once a product requires a laboratory to make the ingredients instead of Mother Nature, it has entered unhealthy territory.

Many of the flavored waters on the market also contain added nutrients, which give us a seemingly valid reason to let our children drink them: *My child will not drink plain water, but at least he will drink this. The B vitamins it supplies makes it like a multivitamin. My child is a picky eater, so at least she gets some nutrients from the flavored water.* We have heard these reasons, and others, time and again from parents and older children justifying their consumption of these beverages, and we understand how confusing it all can be.

A panel of scientists, in a proposed beverage guidance system, has warned against the perceived value of flavored bottled water drinks that have been fortified with essential nutrients. Children can get all the required nutrients from a well-balanced diet, the panel argued. Reaching for one or two vitamins in a drink does not accomplish the goal of eating a varied diet rich in vegetables, fruits, whole grains, low-fat protein, and dairy products.

Other ingredients that may be found in these flavored waters include herbs (yerba mate), noncaloric sweeteners (stevia and erythritol), and taurine. For convenience, you can also get your chemicals in drops to add to your own bottle or glass of water. One brand of these drops contains artificial sweeteners, artificial colors, citric or malic acid, flavors, and preservatives. An alternative? SweetLeaf has a line of flavored stevias that contain only natural flavors without chemicals.

Like flavored milk, juice, and energy drinks, most flavored water contains added sugar. Most flavored water has approximately 13 grams (3¼ teaspoons) of added sugar per serving, and most of us think that a flavored water bottle is one serving size when in fact it is two or more. One popular brand of flavored water has 13 grams (3¼ teaspoons) of sugar per serving but the bottle has 2.5 servings, totaling 32.5 grams of added sugar (8 teaspoons), which is close to that of soda and more sugar than found in a cup of juice.

Your child needs to drink plain water, not sugar-loaded flavored water, even if it is enhanced with some vitamins. As a treat occasionally, when your child has completed this program, you can reach for a flavored water that is free of artificial ingredients, but make sure you let your child drink only an 8-ounce serving, not the entire bottle.

Should Children Drink Tap or Bottled Water?

If you have well water, get it tested to see whether it contains contaminants or microorganisms. If it does, you will need to treat the water appropriately with the help of an expert.

You may also want to invest in a filter that purifies water by reverse osmosis and carbon block filtration. If your well water is clean, offer it to your family. If the water from your tap is town or city water, look into how your community purifies it first before consuming it. You may or may not need to filter it some more. Basically whether you drink tap or filtered water, you're way ahead!

You can find an excellent and reasonably priced water filter at www.JacobsonHealth.com.

When Tea and Coffee Resemble Dessert

Remember the day when a cup of coffee or tea was just that? Today's cafés are a frequent gathering place for children, especially teens and tweens, and they offer coffee and tea in forms that resemble ice cream: iced cappuccinos and iced green tea smoothies. Who can blame our kids for wanting to try them and then becoming addicted?

Children want to be just like grownups from an early age, and drinking coffee is an adult behavior (or at least it used to be) that makes them feel mature. When you look at the age of some children ordering coffee and tea at shops today, they seem to get younger and younger. One National Health and Nutrition Examination Survey study found that from 1988 to 2004 consumption of coffee and tea rose across all ages: from 1 to 2 percent for children two to five years of age; from 1 to 3 percent for children six to eleven years; and from 6 to 9 percent for tweens and teenagers.

Children face the same risks when consuming coffee and tea as they do when drinking other sugary, caffeinated beverages. A study of more than 1,000 children under the age of fifteen showed that those who consumed tea and coffee regularly were at an increased risk of developing type 1 diabetes. In people with type 1 diabetes, the pancreas cannot make enough insulin, so daily injections of insulin are needed. It is much more serious than the increased risk of type 2 diabetes.

We cannot recommend that children consume caffeinated coffee and tea because we don't know the effects of caffeine on growing children. We also do not recommend flavored coffee and tea drinks because of the insane amount of sugar found in them. The sugar in lattes at Starbucks can range from 10 to 38 grams, 10 to 12 grams of added sugar is found in their cappuccinos, 20 to 55 grams in mochas, and a whopping 44 to 81 grams in Frappuccinos. Coolattas at Dunkin' Donuts are no better, with 40 to 87 grams of added sugar depending on the flavor. There are also 10 to 43 grams of sugar in Dunkin' Donuts iced lattes and up to 63 grams of added sugar in hot lattes.

Is Decaffeinated Tea or Coffee Okay for Kids?

We do not recommend any type of coffee for children, whether caffeinated or decaffeinated. When it comes to tea, decaffeinated tea in moderation is okay as long as you choose wisely. Watch out for the added sugar because iced teas can pack a punch—20 or more grams of sugar per cup in some brands.

Also avoid iced tea that is artificially flavored, artificially colored, or artificially sweetened. Look for brands that are brewed from tea leaves. You can always make a homemade batch of caffeine-free herbal tea from tea bags or pouches. They come in a wide variety of flavors and you can sweeten them with stevia, lowering the amount of stevia over time as your child's taste buds recover from having been "sugar bombed."

It's best if your children avoid all coffee and caffeinated tea beverages because of the caffeine and added sugar they contain. Children should focus on getting their recommended daily amount of milk and water first, along with a balanced diet.

Parent Advice on Handling Tantrums

Your children will most likely throw a fit when you take away what they love most, especially when they are addicted to it. You can expect that your children will have outbursts of anger and frustration when they are not allowed to drink their favorite drink or eat their favorite sweet snack. Preparing your child is the best thing you can do to prevent an outburst. Children are smart and we tend to underestimate how much they can comprehend complex issues. Sit down with your children and discuss the reasons for your decision to remove sugar from their diet. Follow this with a detailed list of what they will be required to do during the program and the consequences that will ensue if the rules are not followed.

Very young children (two to three years old) may not be able to understand what is going on; they just know that they feel confused and lousy when sugar is removed from their diet and they act out because of it. It is best to stay home or at least limit trips to the store during the emotionally charged days to allow young children the space to express themselves without the additional burden of having to behave in public. The time it will take to settle down will differ for each child. It depends on how much sugar they consume to begin with plus the individual effects this sugar has on them personally. Know that there is an end in sight and that we have specifically created the *Beat Sugar Addiction Now for Kids* program to minimize physical and emotional responses to coming off of sugar.

Preschool- and elementary-aged children could also use a break from the responsibility of having to behave themselves in public during the first several days after you remove their favorite beverage or food. Taking them to the grocery store right after you stopped giving them their drink of choice is asking for trouble. If you must grocery shop with them, avoid the aisles that have the food or beverage that you removed from their diet.

When tweens or teenagers throw a fit, send them to their room to work it out themselves. They will need extra sleep during periods of withdrawal, especially if they are consuming a lot of drinks with added caffeine. Give them a break when appropriate, but don't let them cross the line. Follow the advice discussed previously for easing withdrawal symptoms to lessen the occurrence of outbursts.

Fun and Easy Drink Recipes You Can Make with Your Children

Here are some healthy and delicious alternative drinks you can offer your children, and if you make them together, you'll have greater buy-in and a fun bonding experience.

Homemade flavored water. In a pitcher filled with water and ice, add one or a combination of the following: lemon slices, cucumber slices, orange slices, lime slices, fresh mint leaves, or apple slices. Leave the pitcher on the shelf closest to your children's height in the front of the refrigerator or on the counter where they can reach it easily. Easy access will go a long way in encouraging your children to drink this healthy beverage. It also looks very pretty. As your kids get accustomed to the lack of sweetness over time, their taste buds will once again be able to enjoy the subtle flavors found in this drink.

Homemade fizzy pop. To 8 ounces (235 ml) of seltzer or sparkling water, add 1 ounce of your child's favorite juice (the juice counts toward his daily recommended limit). For extra sparkle, add a slice of orange, lemon, or lime.

N'ice tea. To make homemade iced tea, start by adding any of the following herbal tea bags to boiling water: chamomile, ginger, nettle leaf, lemongrass, or peppermint. Add one tea bag for every cup of tea. You can use one kind or a combination of teas. Our favorite is two nettle leaf tea bags, one ginger tea bag, and one lemongrass tea bag to 1 quart of water. Add 1 teaspoon of honey to 1 quart (1 L) of the tea and let it steep until cool. Pour the cooled tea over ice and 4 cups (950 ml) of cold water, add some mint leaves, if desired, and enjoy. Note: Do not offer mint tea to young children because the flavor is too strong for them. Do not offer chamomile to children with ragweed allergies.

Daily Beverage Intake Form

Write down how much of each of these beverages your children consume in one day. For example, if your children drink ½ cup (120 ml) of juice for breakfast, write ½ cup (120 ml) in the column under breakfast for Juice: 100 percent. Ask your children what they drank as soon as they get home from school or a play date. You can do this for two to three days and average the amounts to get a more accurate measure.

Beverage	Breakfast	Morning	Lunch	Afternoon	Dinner	After dinner
Water						
Juice: 100 percent						
Juice drink						
Milk						
Flavored milk						
Soda						
Diet soda						
Energy drink						
Flavored water						
Sports drink						
Coffee						
Tea and iced tea						

Coffee and Tea Goal Sheet

Create a calendar, use the one in your home, or download one from the Internet.

Directions: Children earn 5 points each day they reduce the amount of coffee and caffeinated tea they consume. Deduct 5 points each time they drink more than their daily allotment of coffee and caffeinated tea. Fill in the calendar with starting amounts and daily goals and post it on the refrigerator so they can see what is expected each day.

Step 1: Eliminate caffeinated tea

Each week, replace 1 cup (235 ml) of hot or cold caffeinated tea with water. Continue to eliminate 1 cup (235 ml) of hot or cold caffeinated tea a week until zero is reached.

Step 2: Eliminate coffee

Reduce coffee drinks by one a week and replace with water until zero is reached.

The maximum points children earn depends on where they started. Determine their maximum points by multiplying the number of days it will take to reduce their current caffeinated tea and coffee consumption until goal. For example, if they currently consume two coffee drinks a day and one iced tea, it will take them 3 weeks (21 days) to reach the goal. They would earn 5 points for each of the 21 days, for a total of 105 points.

To determine whether they reached their goal, multiply 105 points by 80 percent (0.8) = 84 points, 60 percent (0.6) × 105 = 63 points. Now you can determine whether they achieved the goal, i.e., 84 to 105 points, got second place if points fell in the 63 to 83 point range, or need to try again if they scored under 63 points.

Made goal: If they earn 80 to 100 percent of their points.

Second place: If they earn 60 to 79 percent of their points, they should follow the program until they are able to avoid coffee and tea at least 6 or 7 days a week.

Try again: If they earn fewer than 60 percent of their points, they should go back to whichever step is necessary and continue until they are able to avoid coffee and caffeinated tea 6 or 7 days a week.

I will earn _____ for reaching my goal.

Flavored Milk Goal Sheet

Create a calendar, use the one in your home, or download one from the Internet.

Directions: Give 5 points or one sticker (for younger children) each time your children reduce flavored milk outside the home during step 1, drink diluted milk during step 2 (if you are following this optional step), and consume the reduced amount during step 3, until they reach their goal. Deduct 5 points when they drink more than their daily flavored milk allotment. Fill in the calendar with starting amounts and daily goals and post it on the refrigerator so your children can see what is expected of them each day.

Daily milk or milk alternative goals for children:

2 to 3 years old: 2 cups (470 ml) plain milk per day

4 to 8 years old: 2½ cups (570 ml) plain milk per day

9 to 13 years old: 3 cups (700 ml) plain milk per day

14 to 18 years old: 3 cups (700 ml) plain milk per day

Step 1: Reduce chocolate and other flavored milk outside the home by 1 cup (235 ml) or one 6- to 8-ounce (175 to 235 ml) box every four days. Replace the flavored milk they were drinking outside the home with plain milk.

Step 2 (optional): Dilute flavored milk by 2 oz (60 ml) on day one and 1 oz (28 ml) on day 3 until your children react to the difference in taste. Start step 3 with the diluted milk that your children tolerate.

Plain milk to flavored milk ratio:

2 oz to 6 oz (60 to 175 ml) (day 1)

3 oz to 5 oz (90 to 150 ml) (day 2)

4 oz to 4 oz (120 to 120 ml) (day 3)

5 oz to 3 oz (150 to 90 ml) (day 4)

6 oz to 2 oz (175 to 60 ml) (day 5)

Step 3: Reduce the amount of flavored milk your children drink (diluted or undiluted) by 1 oz (28 ml) for younger children and 2 oz (60 ml) for older children at each serving until your children no longer drink any flavored milk. Replace the flavored milk with plain low-fat milk until your children reach their daily goal for dairy (or dairy alternative).

continued on next page

Flavored Milk Goal Sheet (continued)

The maximum points they can earn depends on where they started. Determine the maximum points by multiplying the number of days it will take your children to reduce their current flavored milk consumption until they reach goal. If your young child currently consumes 3 cups (700 ml) of flavored milk a day (one at each meal including one at school) he or she would earn 60 points. It would take 4 days of 5 points a day to stop drinking flavored milk at school, plus it would take him or her 8 days to eliminate the flavored milk (1 oz/day reduction) at lunch and dinner (5 points × 4 = 20 for eliminating chocolate milk outside the home, plus 8 × 5 = 40 to eliminate chocolate milk at home, for a grand total of 60 points).

Made goal: If they earn 80 to 100 percent of their points.

Second place: If they earn 60 to 79 percent of their points, they should follow the program until they are able to avoid flavored milk at least 6 to 7 days a week.

Try again: If they earn fewer than 60 percent of their points, they should go back to whichever step is necessary and continue until they are able to avoid flavored milk 6 to 7 days a week.

I will earn _____ for reaching my goal.

Flavored Water and Sports Drink Goal Sheet

Create a calendar, use the one in your home, or download one from the Internet.

Directions: Give 5 points or one sticker (for younger children) each time your children drink water and not a sports drink during an activity and each time they reduce and replace flavored water and sports drinks with plain water. Deduct 5 points each time they drink more than the daily allotment of flavored water or sports drinks and each time they consume a sports drink during an activity (unless medically necessary). Fill in the calendar with starting amounts and daily goals and post it on the refrigerator so your children can see what is expected each day.

Step 1: Bring water to sports events.

Step 2: Reduce and replace sports drinks. Reduce the amount of sports drinks your children consume daily by ½ cup (120 ml) a day until they reach zero and replace with ½ cup (120 ml) water.

Step 3: Reduce and replace flavored water. Reduce flavored water in your children's diet by ½ cup (120 ml) a day until they reach zero and replace with ½ cup (120 ml) water.

Maximum points they can earn depends on where they started. Determine maximum points by multiplying the number for days it will take your child to reduce their current sports drink and flavored water consumption until they reach the goal. If your child currently drinks 1 sports drink and 2 flavored waters a day plus they bring sports drinks to soccer games they would earn a maximum of 35 points: 2 days x 5 points to stop daily sports drinks (½ cup [120 ml] reduction a day), plus 4 days × 5 points (½ cup [120 ml] reduction a day) to stop daily flavored water, plus if they brought water and no sports drinks to soccer that week, they would earn another 5 points.

Made goal: If they earn 80 to 100 percent of their points.

Second place: If they earn 60 to 79 percent of their points, they should follow the program until they are able to avoid flavored water and sports drinks at least 6 to 7 days a week.

Try again: If they earn less than 60 percent of their points, they should go back to whichever step is necessary and continue until they are able to avoid flavored water and sports drinks 6 to 7 days a week.

I will earn _____ for reaching my goal.

Soda and Energy Drink Goal Sheet

Create a calendar, use the one in your home, or download one from the Internet.

Directions: Give 5 points or one sticker (for younger children) each time they meet daily soda and energy drink reduction goals during steps 2 and 3. Deduct 5 points each time they consume more soda and energy drinks than their daily allotment. Fill in the calendar with starting amounts and daily goals and post it on the refrigerator so you can see what is expected each day.

Step 1: Prepare the house by throwing away soda and energy drinks or do not buy any more and consume what is left in the house.

Step 2: Reduce decaffeinated soda consumption by one can or one (8 oz [235 ml]) glass every four days until they aren't drinking it anymore.

Step 3: Reduce their intake of caffeinated soda or energy drinks by one drink (1 can or 8 ounces [235 ml]) a week until they aren't drinking it anymore.

The maximum points they can earn depends on where they started. Determine maximum points by multiplying the amount for days it will take your children to reduce their current soda and energy drink consumption until they reach the goal. For example, if your children drinks three cans of caffeinated soda and one energy drink a day, it would take 3 weeks to reach the goal for a maximum of 105 points (21 days × 5 = 105).

Made goal: If they earn 80 to 100 percent of their points.

Second place: If they earn 60 to 79 percent of their points, they should follow the program until they are able to avoid soda and energy drinks at least 6 to 7 days a week.

Try again: If they earn fewer than 60 percent of their points, they should go back to whichever step is necessary and continue until they are able to avoid soda and energy drinks 6 to 7 days a week.

I will earn _____ for reaching my goal.

Juice Goal Sheet

Create a calendar, use the one in your home, or download one from the Internet.

Directions: Give 5 points or one sticker (for younger children) each time your children drink 100 percent juice in step 1 and 2 and consume their reduced daily amount in step 3 until they reach their goal. Deduct 5 points when they drink juice drinks or consume more than their daily juice allotment. Fill in the calendar with starting amounts and daily goals and post it on the refrigerator so your children can see what is expected each day.

Daily 100 percent juice intake goal by age:

2 to 3 years: 4 oz (120 ml)

4 to 6 years: 6 oz (175 ml)

7 to 13 years: 8 oz (235 ml)

14 to 18 years: 12 oz (350 ml)

Step 1: Replace your children's juice drink with 100 percent juice.

Step 2 (optional): Dilute 100 percent juice by replacing 1 oz (28 ml) juice with 1 oz (28 ml) water until tolerance.

Step 3: Reduce the amount of juice your children drink by 2 oz (60 ml) a day for children under 7 and 4 oz (120 ml) a day for children 7 years and older.

Step 4: Reduce the number of boxes that they drink by one every three days until the goal is met.

The maximum points they can earn depends on where they started. Determine the maximum points by multiplying the amount of days it will take your children to reduce their current juice consumption until they reach the goal.

For example, if your children currently drink two juice boxes plus 8 oz (235 ml) of juice per day, the maximum points they can earn is 70 if you took the following steps:

☐ You switched their juice from juice-ade to 100 percent juice, which they drank for 3 days (15 points) before diluting it.

☐ Next, you diluted their 8 oz (235 ml) glass of juice in the morning until they noticed (3 days of diluting × 5 = 15 points).

☐ Their total daily amount allowed is 4 oz (120 ml), so it took you 2 days (10 points) to lower the amount to 4 oz (120 ml).

☐ Then, you focused on eliminating the juice boxes, which took 6 days (30 points).

Juice Goal Sheet (continued)

Made goal: If they earn 80 to 100 percent of their points.

Second place: If they earn 60 to 79 percent of their points, they should follow the program until they are able to limit their 100 percent juice intake at least 6 to 7 days a week.

Try again: If they earn fewer than 60 percent of their points, they should go back to whichever step is necessary and continue until they are able to limit their 100 percent juice intake 6 to 7 days a week.

I will earn _____ for reaching my goal.

Chapter 3

Step 2: Revamp Breakfast

Start your children off the right way to avoid sugar highs and lows

Now that your children have reduced their intake of sugar-sweetened beverages, you are ready to begin step 2—revamping their breakfast. Many children start their day eating toaster cakes, sugar-sweetened cereal, breakfast bars, or doughnuts. Although there are healthier alternatives, most children begin their day eating nothing better than candy in disguise with vitamins added for good measure.

Prescription for Revamping Breakfast

The following prescription will help you give your child's breakfast a makeover while limiting the disruption and pushback that may occur. What children eat for breakfast sets the stage for their entire day: begin with a breakfast full of sugar and they are off on a roller-coaster ride of sugar highs and lows with all the accompanying mood swings.

Create a calendar for your children with the points they will earn by referring to the "Revamp Breakfast Goal Sheet" at the end of the chapter.

WEEK 1

Provide a healthy source of protein at breakfast (approximately 6 to 12 g) for your children.
If they are eating an unhealthy source of protein (regular bacon, beef sausages, or ham—see below for healthy versions of these proteins), switch to any of the healthier versions listed below and add it to their breakfast routine:

- Eggs (1): scrambled, boiled, baked, poached, or egg salad
- Sausage (2 links): turkey or chicken sausage

- Seeds (½ to 1 oz), nuts, and nut butter (1 to 2 tablespoons [16 to 32 g]), such as peanut butter, almond butter, sunflower seed butter, or any other nut butter with no added sugar
- Dairy: low- or nonfat milk (8 oz [235 ml]), yogurt (6 to 8 oz [170 to 230 g] with no more than 23 grams of sugars per 8-oz [230 g] serving), cheese (1½ oz [43 g] of hard cheese), or cottage cheese (1 cup [225 g])
- Bacon (2 slices): turkey bacon or nitrite-free bacon (limit to once a week)
- Meat (2 slices or 1 to 2 ounces [28 to 55 g]): sliced turkey, chicken, or ham (free of monosodium glutamate [MSG], nitrates, and nitrites). Note: Applegate Farms makes great sausage, sliced meat, and bacon products free of nitrates, nitrites, and MSG. Many of their products are also organic.

▶ *Note: A child younger than four years should eat half the serving size and a child older than fourteen can eat twice the serving size.*

WEEK 2

Add a serving of fresh fruit to your children's breakfast. You can also serve a glass of juice (½ to 1 cup [120 to 235 ml] a day), but that is optional. You may want to save their juice for later in the day or give them a couple of ounces of juice mixed with 6 oz (175 ml) of water. A great rule for children to follow is to eat a fruit or vegetable at every meal and one at snack time. Because most breakfasts do not contain vegetables, unless an omelet is being prepared, serve fruit with each breakfast. If you do not have access to fresh fruit, do the best you can with the following information:

- Fresh fruit is best.
- Eat a variety of colors.
- If you choose canned fruit or a fruit cup, make sure it does not have added sweeteners. Avoid varieties that are packed in light or heavy syrups. Select those packed in water or fruit juice instead.
- For pureed fruit like applesauce, look for varieties that have no added sugar.

- Do not serve fruit strips, gummy fruit chews, fruit leather, or any other processed fruit item. They contain too much sugar and little to no fiber.
- Dried fruit is high in sugar, so do not serve it as often as whole fruit. Make sure you serve appropriate servings—about half that of whole fruit (¼ cup [40 g]).
- Use these guidelines for fruit serving sizes:
    - 1 small banana (6 inches [15 cm])
    - 1 small apple, pear, orange, or peach
    - ½ cup (75 g) cut-up fruit, berries, or grapes
    - 4-oz (75 g) fruit cup or applesauce containers (no sugar added)
    - ½ cup (75 g) mandarin oranges (only fruit-juice sweetened)
    - ¼ cup raisins or other dried fruit

▶ **Note:** *A child younger than four should eat half of this serving and a child older than fourteen can eat twice the serving size.*

WEEKS 3 AND 4

Switch from processed to whole grains and provide one or two servings of whole grains for breakfast. Take a couple of weeks to replace sweet breakfast items with low-sugar, whole-grain items. For example, offer your children a new cereal to replace their favorite sugary item. Once you have switched the cereal, work on replacing toaster cakes, cinnamon rolls, white bagels, or other sugary breakfast treats. Continue until you have replaced all the sugary breakfast options with healthy whole grains.

These weeks will be the most challenging because chances are your child eats a breakfast high in sugar and these foods are tasty, are heavily marketed as fun, and come in crazy colors and shapes. We promise you, and research supports this, that your children will like the taste of whole grains; it just takes a while for their taste buds to adjust, so you need to stick with it until that occurs.

A younger child should eat one serving of whole grains (1 piece of toast, ½ cup [117 g] of oatmeal, or 1 cup [225 g] of cold cereal); an older child may eat two servings. The magic number for this step is four: purchase breakfast items with 4 grams of sugar or less per serving. Replace the following unhealthy options with the healthy whole-grain versions.

You may also want to try other whole grains that are tasty and may be unfamiliar to you, such as spelt, kamut, rye berries, amaranth, millet, quinoa, and buckwheat.

Healthy Grains versus Unhealthy Grains

Healthy option	Unhealthy option
Whole-grain hot cereal with no more than 1 teaspoon (4 g) of sugar	Hot cereal with added sugar or made with processed grains
Oatmeal made with steel-cut oats, rolled oats, or groats, with no sugar	Oatmeal with more than 1 teaspoon (4 g) of sugar
Grits made from whole-grain grits	Hominy grits, corn grits, hominy
Other whole-grain hot cereal made with brown rice, quinoa, bulgur wheat, or millet	Cream of wheat made with wheat farina
*You may add 1 teaspoon (5 g) of brown sugar or maple syrup and sliced fruit for sweetness to the items listed above if they have no added sugar in them.	
Whole-grain bread. The first ingredient needs to be "whole": whole wheat, whole rye, whole barley, whole oats, brown rice, white whole wheat, whole durum, or whole bulgur *Pumpernickel bread is a rye bread. Choose varieties made with rye berries or whole rye flour. *White whole wheat bread is now on the market. Make sure the first ingredient is white whole wheat. *You may add 1 teaspoon (4 g) of jam to bread.	Bread made with wheat or white flour: white, rye, cinnamon, English muffins, pita, tortilla, pumpernickel
Bagel made with whole wheat, whole oat, whole rye, or white whole wheat as the first ingredient	Bagels made with wheat or white flour (white, raisin, pumpernickel, poppy, sesame, onion, everything bagel)
Whole-grain cereal with minimal sugar added. Choose brands with 4 grams or less of sugar per cup of cereal.	Cold cereal: sugar sweetened, ready to eat
Homemade whole-grain toast with 1 teaspoon (4 g) of jam and/or nut and seed butters	Toaster cakes
Waffles and pancakes made with whole wheat or other whole grains like buckwheat *You may add 1 teaspoon (4 g) of pure maple syrup and sliced fruit or try topping with yogurt	Waffles and pancakes made with white flour
French toast made with whole-grain bread	French toast made with white bread
Put ¼ cup (40 g) of dried fruit (raisins, cranberries, cherries) in a baggie with nuts, seeds, and 1 cup (100 g) of dried whole-grain cereal or roasted oats	Breakfast bars or granola bars
Replace with any whole-grain option listed above	Doughnuts, coffee cake, breakfast rolls

Putting Together a Healthy Breakfast

Breakfast is the meal that sets the mood for the entire day. If your children start their day with a healthy breakfast low in sugar, they will have the energy they need to be productive during their morning activities and will be less likely to crave sugar mid-morning or later in the day. Here are some of the other benefits children experience when they start their day eating a healthy breakfast. They will

- Do better in school
- Have better hand-eye coordination
- Manage their weight better
- Be more likely to engage in physical activity
- Have a healthier diet overall

You don't have to be a chef or nutritionist to provide a healthy breakfast. Just remember that there are three essential components to any healthy breakfast: a whole grain, a protein, and a fruit. Whole grains are a great source of energy, nutrients, and fiber that fill up your children's stomach so that they feel full for a longer period of time. The protein at breakfast provides essential body-building nutrients and helps even out blood sugar levels after eating. Last, whole fruit supplies vitamins and fiber along with water and a lot less sugar than juice delivers. We have provided a list of healthy breakfast foods for your children to choose from at the end of this chapter. (See "Build Your Breakfast.")

A healthy breakfast = whole grain + protein + fruit

How to Make Breakfast in No Time

No matter how much time you have in the morning, you can throw together a healthy breakfast for your child. We have listed healthy suggestions that you can make in as little as five minutes as well as options that take a little more time for those mornings when you are not rushing to get your children out the door.

WHEN YOU HAVE 5 MINUTES OR LESS

- Sandwiches: Start with whole-grain bread or a whole-grain bagel, add 1 to 2 tablespoons (16 to 32 g) nut butter or sunflower seed butter and 1 teaspoon (7 g) jam (optional), or a slice of sandwich meat with low-fat mayonnaise or mustard. Add a piece of fruit and water.

- Fruit-cheese wraps: On a whole-grain 6-inch (15 cm) tortilla or a large tortilla cut in half, spread low-fat cream cheese and have your child select a fruit to sprinkle on top (raisins, dried cranberries, bananas, peach slices). Roll and go.

- Banana–nut butter wraps: On a whole-grain 6-inch (15 cm) tortilla or a large tortilla cut in half, spread 1 to 2 tablespoons (16 to 32 g) nut butter or sunflower seed butter. Place a peeled banana in the middle, roll, and go.

- Yogurt, whole-grain cereal, and a piece of fruit: Put some berries in a plastic bag with dry cereal. Your children can add it to the yogurt in the car as you drive them to school or practice.

- Yogurt smoothies: Add ½ cup (75 g) frozen fruit to ½ cup (4 oz [115 g]) plain yogurt and ½ cup (120 ml) low-fat milk. Blend in the blender until all the ingredients are mixed (add more milk if it is too thick). Pour into a glass and enjoy. Serve with a handful of dried whole-grain cereal.

- Whole-grain cereal: Add a cup of milk and sliced fruit on top.

- Whole-grain waffles: Top with nut butter or yogurt and sprinkle with fruit.

- Whole-grain English muffin: Toast and add 1 to 2 oz (28 to 56 g) of cheese and an apple.

- Mix chopped fruit with cottage cheese: Add a piece of toast or dried whole-grain cereal.

WHEN YOU HAVE 10 TO 20 MINUTES

- Eggs and toast: Serve a scrambled, boiled, or poached egg with whole-grain toast and an orange. For a twist, stuff a whole-grain pita pocket with scrambled eggs for a tasty, on-the-go option.

- Whole-grain pancakes: Serve with turkey sausage and apple slices.

- Whole-grain French toast: Combine 2 eggs, ½ cup (120 ml) almond milk or low-fat milk, ¼ teaspoon ground cinnamon, and ¼ teaspoon vanilla extract. Dip a thick piece of whole-grain bread into the egg mixture. Cook in a frying pan with a little bit of butter or transfat-free margarine.

- Homemade oatmeal: You can make a batch of whole-grain oatmeal, also known as steel-cut oats or groats, in 20 to 30 minutes, and reheat in small batches for several days after. Add low-fat milk, ground cinnamon, ½ cup (125 g) no-sugar-added applesauce, and 1 tablespoon (9 g) raisins.

- Omelet: Add 1 tablespoon olive oil to a 12-inch (30 cm) frying pan and place the pan over medium heat. Add chopped onions and peppers, spinach, or other vegetables you have in the refrigerator that your child likes. Whisk 2 eggs with 1 teaspoon (5 ml) water (it is easier to make a two-egg omelet and split it with your child than to make a one-egg omelet). Add to the cooked vegetables. Fold in half when the sides are cooked and it is easy to turn. Add cheese on top, if you like, and serve.

- Individual frittatas: Preheat the oven to 325°F (170°C), gas mark 3. Sauté diced bell peppers and onions in 1 tablespoon (14 g) olive oil in a frying pan until soft, about 5 to 7 minutes. Remove from the heat. Beat 4 eggs in a bowl and then add ⅓ cup (70 ml) milk (nonfat or low fat) to the egg mixture. Add sautéed veggies and stir. Pour immediately into a greased cupcake pan, filling the cups three-quarters full. Bake for 15 minutes. Serve with a piece of whole-grain toast. You can make enough frittatas for two or three days and reheat before serving.

Beat Sugar Addiction Now for Kids

The Truth about Carbohydrates

Carbohydrates, the body's primary source of energy, provide the body with sugar. Sugar can exist in a simple form that is easily absorbed and raises blood sugar levels quickly, like that found in white bread, for example, or it can be bundled up into complex carbohydrates known as starches, which are harder to break down as long as they are whole grain and not refined. Examples of complex carbohydrates include steel-cut oats, whole wheat bread, bulgur, and quinoa. Whole grains contain the germ, bran, and endosperm and are harder to digest than simple processed flour items that contain only the endosperm of the grain.

When your child eats whole grains, nutrients are released slowly over time because your child's body has to work at breaking down the complex carbohydrates into sugar molecules. Processed grain, on the other hand, releases sugar into the bloodstream in one giant flood, which causes a spike in blood sugar levels just like if your child ate pure sugar.

How high blood sugar levels rise after a food is eaten is called the glycemic index of that food. Foods that have a high glycemic index cause a high rise in blood sugar after being eaten and include ice cream, soda, dried fruit, and processed grains like white bread and cornflakes. Low-glycemic-index foods include vegetables, whole grains, milk, nuts, and vegetables. To find the glycemic index on more than one hundred foods, go to www.health.harvard.edu/newsweek/Glycemic_index_and_glycemic_load_for_100_foods.htm.

We appreciate that the entire issue of sugar and carbohydrates can be confusing. Carbohydrates were the latest "villain" that nutritionists were fighting over. It was just recently that we got over a low-carb phase, during which we were led to believe that carbohydrates were not healthy and caused weight gain. We now know that carbohydrates in general are not the bad guy, but some types of carbohydrates are unhealthy in excess.

Here are the facts:

- Kids should consume 50 to 60 percent of their calories as carbohydrates.
- Complex carbohydrates, also known as starches, are part of a healthy diet if they come from whole-grain sources and not from refined grains.
- Children should eat healthy sources of simple carbohydrates (just a fancy word for sugars). Simple sugars are found in many healthy foods like milk products (lactose), fruits (fructose), and grains (glucose).
- Limit foods with refined sugar (added sugar) and refined grains (processed grains). You will need to look at the ingredients list to search for added sugar. These are some of the names that sugar takes on:

  – anhydrous dextrose
  – brown sugar
  – cane juice
  – confectioners' or powdered sugar
  – corn syrup
  – corn syrup solids
  – crystal dextrose
  – dextrose
  – evaporated corn sweetener
  – fructose
  – fruit juice concentrate
  – fruit nectar
  – glucose
  – high-fructose corn syrup
  – honey
  – invert sugar
  – lactose
  – liquid fructose
  – malt syrup
  – maltose
  – maple syrup
  – molasses
  – nectars (e.g., peach nectar, pear nectar)
  – pancake syrup
  – raw sugar
  – sucrose
  – sugar
  – sugar cane juice
  – granulated (white) sugar

Symptoms of a Sugar Disorder

Let's follow the path of these two boys: Ben starts his day with scrambled eggs, whole-grain toast, and a peach. Jon starts his day with a glass of juice and a toaster cake that he eats while running to the bus. Ben's body has 4 grams (1 teaspoon) of simple sugar to deal with while Jon's body has 40 grams (4 teaspoons) of sugar to digest and metabolize. Because Jon's breakfast has little to no fiber or protein, all that sugar is going to be absorbed quickly.

Ben's body will absorb the sugar in his meal slowly over a period of time because of the fiber in the whole grains and the protein in the eggs. Ben will feel fuller longer; his body will get a steady release of sugar for energy to last him until his next meal or snack, and he will be able to concentrate in school.

Jon, on the other hand will have a spike in his blood sugar level because of the huge load of sugar that was present in his meal. His pancreas will do its best to handle the sugar load, but it was not designed to handle that much sugar at once. The sugar in his blood will drop quickly to either a normal range and he will feel hungry shortly after breakfast, or his sugar level will drop below normal and create a state of hypoglycemia (low blood sugar). Either way, he will crave more sugar soon after breakfast. If Jon eats like this day after day, chances are he will begin to have a problem regulating his blood sugar levels because of the stress the sugar has on his pancreas; the sugar levels will either get too high (diabetes) or too low (hypoglycemia).

If you sense that your children are having a problem with their sugar levels (see the "Sugar Disorder Checklist" at the end of the chapter), look for the following signs and always check with their pediatrician if you have any concerns to rule out other dangerous causes of their symptoms. Unfortunately, most nonholistic physicians are not yet familiar with the common low blood sugar problems seen with sweets (only with severe coma caused by low blood sugar in children on insulin).

Symptoms of low blood sugar (possibly hypoglycemia) can include the following:

- Hunger pain/stomachache, extreme hunger
- Severe sugar cravings
- Shakiness or tremors
- Moodiness or crankiness
- Learning and behavioral disorders
- Nervousness
- Sweating
- Pale gray skin color
- Headache

- Dizziness
- Sleepiness
- Confusion
- Difficulty speaking
- Anxiety
- Weakness
- Blurred vision
- Unconsciousness and seizures, when severe

Symptoms of high blood sugar (possibly diabetes) can include the following:

- Increased urination
- Increased thirst
- Black velvety discoloration to the neck and skin folds
- Hypertension

- Increased hunger
- Fatigue
- Slow-healing sores
- Recurrent infections
- Blurred vision

▶ **Note:** *Some children experience no symptoms with high blood sugar.*

Parent Tips and Tricks

You may run into the following issues when revamping your children's breakfast. Below are solutions, advice, and information to encourage your children to eat whole-grain products, limit their exposure to ads promoting unhealthy food, and set rules about buying unhealthy breakfast items at fast-food restaurants and doughnut shops.

Q: How do I get through the transition time when my children are upset and screaming about not getting their favorite cereal, toaster cake, or doughnut?
A: Your children will most likely go through a period when they are very angry about not having their favorite breakfast foods. Try the following techniques:

- Reassure your children that not having the cereal of their choice is just for now and that at the end of the program they will be able to have their favorite treat now and again (no more often than one to two times a month, but they don't need to know that now). Chances are, when you get them accustomed to a healthy breakfast, their desire to eat the junky stuff will lessen or go away.
- Let your children know that you hear their frustration, anger, and pain. When they tell you that they are upset, repeat back to them, "I know you are upset about not having your favorite cereal. It must not feel good to you right now, but it will get better." Acknowledging their feelings is important, but it doesn't mean that you have to do anything about it.
- Try to remove their favorite items on the weekend or when you have plenty of time in the morning. You want to avoid having a time constraint that leads to them missing the bus or a game or practice because they are pitching a fit. Being pressured with time by needing to leave the house will worsen an already stressful situation.

- Remove one item at a time instead of jumping in and taking away their cereal, toaster cake, doughnut, and other "candy in disguise." Start by switching their favorite cereal with a whole-grain option. When they are used to that, replace their toaster cake with whole-grain toast. Continue this until you have replaced their usual sweet fare with healthy options. Make sure you don't take away one unhealthy item and introduce another unhealthy one in its place.
- Set up a system of rewards as discussed in previous chapters.
- Try some of the same techniques discussed in the previous chapter to help them manage their withdrawal symptoms:
  - Make sure they get enough rest.
  - Let them run off their frustrations by exercising daily.
  - Make sure they go outside daily for air and sunshine.
  - Keep them hydrated with lots of water.
  - Allow them the space and time to vent.
  - Do not engage in their frustration and anger; remain calm for your child.

Q: What if my child refuses to eat whole-grain products?
A: Replacing processed grain with unprocessed grain is, well, a process and not one that children like very much. If your children are used to only processed grains, they will most likely resist the different taste, appearance, and texture of whole grains, so take it slow in the beginning. When making pasta, substitute one-quarter of the amount you are making with whole-grain noodles. Increase the amount of whole-grain pasta that you add over time until you reach 100 percent whole grain. If the color of whole-grain pasta immediately turns your child off, hide it in a thick sauce; tomato-based sauces work well. This same

technique works for rice, hot cereal, and cold cereal—add more whole-grain cereal and less sugary cereal each day until you have switched them over.

Bread is a different story; it is harder to trick your kids into eating whole-grain bread because of its typical whole-grain appearance—brown versus white, a hearty texture, and visible flecks of whole grain in the slices. Many parents have resorted to buying the new "white whole-grain" bread available on the market. This bread is supposed to be made from albino white wheat instead of the traditional red wheat that most wheat products are made from. Although these white whole-grain products sound like a great idea, consider the following issues:

- Many white whole-grain products contain more processed wheat flour than whole grain, and some contain no white whole grain at all.
- There are many chemicals added to make the white whole-grain product appear, feel, and taste like regular white bread.
- Eating processed bread, even the white whole-grain varieties, does not teach your child to enjoy the taste and texture of other hearty whole-grain products.
- White whole-grain bread is mostly about tricky marketing and often does not hold up to the criteria of "whole" grain as the first ingredient.

Most likely you will need to resort to some sort of bribery to get your kids to eat whole-grain breads. Try the sticker method discussed in chapter 1 for younger children and the point system for older kids. Your goal is to get them to try whole-grain items because once they get used to the whole-grain taste and texture, it will no longer be a daily fight. Once you have switched your child over to eating whole grains, do not go back to buying processed grains at home. Kids like, and will eat, what they are accustomed to eating.

Q: What do I do when my child just wants what she sees on TV?

A: By the time children enter first grade in the United States, they will have watched television an equivalent of three school years' worth of time, with 40,000 advertisements a year, half of which are for food. Of those for food, 98 percent are for unhealthy food. By the time they are eighteen, they will have watched 200,000 commercials. If that isn't brainwashing, we don't know what is.

Training your child to mute advertisements when they come on will lessen their exposure to these messages promoting unhealthy food and beverages. These ads affect the choices that your child makes at the store and the kitchen table, which is why manufacturers spend millions creating these ads. They also prompt your child while watching TV to eat what they see being advertised, which can lead to your child overeating.

If you watch most ads for toaster cakes, you see kids dancing, smiling, and being joyful, and the subtext is "if we are good parents, we will buy food that makes our kids happy." These subtle messages have worked their way into many parents' minds as they buy into the concept that eating is about fun and making our children happy. It isn't; eating a healthy diet is about being together as a family while everyone nourishes his or her body. The fun comes from the personal interactions your child has while helping prepare meals and by eating meals together as a family. If you focus on giving your children only food that makes them happy, you will be training them to eat foods high in sugar, processed grains, and fat, also known as junk food but sold as healthy breakfast alternatives.

Q: How do I break the habit of stopping at doughnut shops or the drive-throughs?

A: Before your children leave the house in the morning, make sure they eat a healthy breakfast. If your children are not hungry when you pass the golden arches or the doughnut shop, they will be less likely to scream for you to stop. Also make sure that you have healthy snacks on hand in the car so that you can thwart any mid-morning or mid-afternoon cravings for sweets. Apples and almonds, homemade trail mix, and whole-grain pretzel sticks will help do the trick.

Sit down with your children at the beginning of step 2 and discuss that you will no longer be stopping for fast food, doughnuts, or other sweet treats available from drive-throughs. Let them know the reason why: these foods prevent them from playing their best, and they are not foods that make them grow up big and strong. Preparing and informing your children helps get them involved and sets their expectations before you leave the house. Let them know that this won't be forever and that once they have completed the program, you can decide whether you want to make these stops a once- or twice-a-month activity. We don't recommend forbidding them entirely, just setting reasonable limits and sticking to them. It is easy to have bad habits sneak back in to daily routines, so be aware and keep on top of the amount of time you stop to buy these sugary treats.

When you do stop, make sure you look at the number of grams of sugar the items contain, because they can vary widely. For example, a glazed doughnut at Dunkin' Donuts has 12 grams of sugar, a glazed stick 23 grams, and a blue-berry crumb doughnut a whopping 52 grams of sugar. Each restaurant has the nutrition information of its products available on its website and it should also have this information available at the restaurant, but you need to ask for it.

Healthy Breakfast Options

Cereals and toaster cakes are often just candy in disguise. Let's take a look at the sugar content of some major breakfast items.

Food	Sugar per serving
Pop-Tarts	Approximately 18 g (4½ teaspoons)
Cap'n Crunch cereal	12 g (3 teaspoons)
Quaker Instant Oatmeal Dinosaur Eggs	16 g (4 teaspoons)
Dunkin' Donuts apple crumb doughnut	49 g (12¼ teaspoons)
Peanut M&Ms	27 g (6¼ teaspoons)

Before you go to the grocery store to look for tasty whole-grain options to offer your child for breakfast, be prepared. We don't want you to feel overwhelmed when you hit the cereal aisle and are faced with hundreds of choices for cold cereal alone. Shopping has become an overwhelming task for many of us, and even we, as doctors, get tripped up now and again. Reading food labels can be tricky, but if you know a few things you will become a pro in no time. Also, teach your child how to read labels. Refer to the "Breakfast Spy Facts" sheet at the end of this chapter.

SHOPPING TIPS
- 1 teaspoon of sugar = 4 grams
- There should be no more than 4 grams of sugar per serving on the Nutrition Facts label on the package for grain items that you serve at breakfast: bread, cereal, waffles, or pancakes.

- The first item on the ingredients list for grains should be "whole grain": whole wheat, whole corn, or whole rye, for example.
- If sugar is first, second, or third on the ingredients list, find a healthier option.
- There should be at least 2 grams of fiber per serving for grain items 80 calories and under and 3 grams for items over 80 calories.
- If you find an item with low sugar content, check for sugar alcohol (sorbitol) or artificial sweetener (sucralose) in the ingredients list. If it is there, choose another low-sugar option without these ingredients.

We provide a list of whole-grain items that meet the criteria of 4 grams of sugar or less per serving in the appendix.

BRAND BREAKFAST ITEMS

Here are some items that we found that are low in sugar and made with whole grain. The list is not complete as ingredients can change, new items are added often, and it does not include store brands.

Cold cereals: General Mills Cheerios (original flavor only), General Mills Kix (original flavor), General Mills Wheaties, Kellogg's Corn Flakes (they are low in fiber), Post Shredded Wheat (original), Post Shredded Wheat 'n Bran, Post Grape-Nuts, Cascadian Farm Organic Multi Grain Squares, Cascadian Farm Organic Purely O's, Kashi 7 Whole Grain Puffs, Kashi 7 Whole Grain Nuggets, Uncle Sam Original Cereal, New Morning Oatios Original, Nature's Path Organic Flax Plus, Barbara's Shredded Wheat, Weetabix

Hot cereal: Quaker Instant Oatmeal Original, Quaker Oats Old Fashioned, Quaker Steel Cut Oats, McCann's Quick Cooking Irish Oatmeal, The Silver Palate Thick and Rough Oatmeal, Bob's Red Mill Organic Scottish Oatmeal, Bob's Red Mill Organic Brown Rice Farina Creamy Rice Hot Cereal, Bob's Red Mill 7-, 8-, or 10-Grain Hot Cereal, Bob's Red Mill 5-Grain Rolled Whole Grain Hot Cereal, Bob's Red Mill Gluten Free Mighty Tasty Hot Cereal

Waffles: Kashi Waffles 7 Grain, Kashi Waffles Blueberry, Van's Natural Foods Waffles 97 percent Fat Free

Revamp Breakfast Goal Sheet

Make a calendar, use the one in your home, or download one from the Internet.

Directions: Give 5 points or one sticker (for younger children) each time your children eat the following at breakfast: a healthy source of protein (5 points), a whole grain (5 points), and a whole fruit (5 points). Deduct 5 points when your child eats processed grain or sugar-sweetened breakfast items.

Week 1: Add a healthy source of protein at each breakfast.

Week 2: Add a whole fruit at breakfast.

Weeks 3 and 4: Serve 1 to 2 servings of whole grains for breakfast and switch from processed to whole grains.

The maximum points they can earn is 325.

Made goal: Earned 275 to 325 points.

Second place: Earned 200 to 275 points: Keep following the program until your child earns more points.

Try again: Earned fewer than 200 points. Start the month over again.

I will earn _____ for reaching my goal.

Build Your Breakfast

Start your day off strong! Build your own breakfast by choosing one item from each column below.

A healthy breakfast = protein + 1 whole fruit + whole grain

1. Start with protein

☐ Eggs (1)   ☐ Milk (8 oz [235 ml])

☐ Turkey/chicken sausage (2 links)   ☐ Cheese (1½ oz [43 g] hard cheese)

☐ Nitrate-free sliced meat (2 slices or 1 to 2 oz [8 to 16 g])   ☐ Seeds (½ to 1 oz 14 to 28 g])

☐ Yogurt (6 oz [172 g])   ☐ Nuts, nut butter (1 to 2 tbsp [9 to 18 g])

Note: A child younger than 4 would eat half the serving size and a child older than 14 could eat twice the serving size.

2. Add some color with whole fruit

☐ Apple   ☐ Clementine

☐ Unsweetened applesauce   ☐ Fruit salad

☐ Banana   ☐ Peach

☐ Berries   ☐ Pear

☐ Grapes   ☐ Any other whole fruit

☐ Orange

3. Choose a whole grain for energy (no more than 4 grams of sugar per serving)

☐ Oatmeal (½ cup [40 g])   ☐ Whole grain bagels (1 medium)

☐ Farina (½ cup [40 g])   ☐ Whole grain waffles (1 waffle)

☐ Brown rice cereal (1 cup [180 g]) ☐ Whole grain pancakes (2 pancakes)

☐ Breakfast cereal (1 cup [180 g])   ☐ Whole grain French toast (1 piece)

☐ Whole-grain toast (1 piece)

Note: A younger child would eat one serving while an older child may eat two servings.

Sugar Disorder Checklist

Place an X next to each symptom that your children experience and note when they usually occur. For example, you may notice that your child gets headaches two hours after he eats. If symptoms are worrisome or persistent despite cutting out excess sugar, consult your pediatrician. Note: Low blood sugar will not usually be detected by standard testing and is based on symptoms rather than lab tests.

Symptoms of low blood sugar can include the following:

- ☐ Hunger pain/stomachache, extreme hunger
- ☐ Severe sugar cravings
- ☐ Shakiness or tremors
- ☐ Moodiness or being cranky
- ☐ Learning and behavioral disorders
- ☐ Nervousness
- ☐ Sweating
- ☐ Pale gray skin color

- ☐ Headache
- ☐ Dizziness
- ☐ Sleepiness
- ☐ Confusion
- ☐ Difficulty speaking
- ☐ Anxiety
- ☐ Weakness
- ☐ Blurred vision

Symptoms of high blood sugar can include the following:

- ☐ Increased urination
- ☐ Increased thirst
- ☐ Black velvety discoloration to the neck and skin folds
- ☐ Hypertension

- ☐ Increased hunger
- ☐ Fatigue
- ☐ Slow healing sores
- ☐ Recurrent infections
- ☐ Blurred vision

Note: Some children experience no symptoms of high blood sugar.

Breakfast Spy Facts

You can discover whether your breakfast is nutritious or just candy in disguise if you follow the secret decoder facts below:

1. Look for "whole" on grain products as the first ingredient.

2. Make sure there are no more than 4 grams of sugars per serving.

3. Avoid numbers with colors: Blue 1, Blue 2, Red 2, Red 3, Red 40, Green 3, Yellow 5, and Yellow 6.

4. Healthier breakfast foods tend to contain short, rather than long, ingredient lists.

Practice decoding these two types of oatmeal. Are they candy in disguise or a healthy breakfast? You figure it out.

A. Quaker Instant Oatmeal Dinosaur Eggs, Maple N Brown Sugar

16 grams of sugar per serving

Ingredients: Whole grain rolled oats (with oat bran), sugar, dinosaur egg-shaped pieces (sugar, dextrose, partially hydrogenated soybean and/or cottonseed oil, maltodextrin, confectioner's glaze, Magnesium Stearate, soy lecithin [an emulsifier], modified corn starch, Red 40 Lake, Yellow 6 Lake, Yellow 5 Lake, artificial color, Blue 1 Lake, bleached beeswax, carnauba wax, natural and artificial flavors), natural and artificial flavors, bone-shaped pieces (sugar, rice flour, confectioner's glaze, partially hydrogenated cottonseed and soybean oil, cornstarch, dextrin, modified food starch, cellulose gum, carnauba wax, carrageenan, bleached beeswax, artificial color, gum tragacanth, Yellow 5, artificial flavor), natural and artificial flavors (contains wheat, soy, and milk components), salt, calcium carbonate (a source of calcium), guar gum, caramel color, niacinamide (one of the B vitamins), vitamin A palmitate, reduced iron, pyridoxine hydrochloride (one of the B vitamins), riboflavin (one of the B vitamins), thiamin mononitrate (one of the B vitamins), folic acid (one of the B vitamins).

B. Quaker Quick Oats, Rolled

1 gram of sugar per serving

Ingredients: 100 percent natural whole grain Quaker quality rolled oats.

Chapter 4

Step 3: Limit Sweets to One per Day and Enjoy Healthy Snacks

How too many discretionary calories and food-based rewards set your child up for a lifelong sugar addiction

Unhealthy snacking has gotten out of control, with 40 percent of our children's calories coming from products with added sugar and solid fats, also known as junk food. Children with a sugar addiction, or an issue regulating their intake of sugar, do best when they eat more frequently. They do not need more calories; rather, they need the calories that they eat to be spread throughout the day to keep their blood sugar levels in a normal, healthy range. Offering your child healthy snacks, full of the nutrients that provide the body with sustained energy they need without spiking their blood sugar levels, is exactly what is required to break their desire for and dependency on sugar.

Getting Ready to Redo Snacking

Begin this step by determining how many unhealthy snacks your children consume on average every day and what time they eat them: morning, afternoon, and after dinner. Write down every snack they eat and then circle the ones that are unhealthy, whether or not they appear to be high in sugar. Unhealthy snacks include all items that have white flour as their first ingredient or sugar as one of the first three ingredients; salty chips; and all foods that are not a fruit, vegetable, nut, seed, whole grain, low-fat protein, or low-fat dairy product with no added sugar. Overly processed grain items like salty chips and white flour–based snacks act as sugar in your child's body, so you will need to focus on removing all but one unhealthy snack (even if they don't seem to be sweet) in this step.

One healthy snack is all your child needs nutrition-wise mid-morning, after school, and after dinner. When your child is addicted to sugar, no amount of sugar-laden food is ever enough, which is why sugar addicts tend to eat more than they need at snack time, and it's not fruits and vegetables they are bingeing on. Once your children's sugar addiction is under control, their bodies will be able to go back to their normal regulation response: they will be able to stop eating when full and eat when hungry. Before that happens, pay attention to serving sizes to make sure your children are not overeating, especially if they also have a weight issue.

Snack Facts You Need to Know

- For children with a sugar issue, two and a half to three hours is the maximum amount of time they should go without eating.
- In general, babies, toddlers, and preschoolers need three snacks a day and older children need two or three snacks a day.
- Once your children get to school, they may or may not need a mid-morning snack—it depends on the time between breakfast and lunch.
- All children need a mid-afternoon/after-school snack.
- Children need an after-dinner snack if it is more than three hours between dinner and bedtime.
- Your children's individual needs will always trump the rules or suggestions. If they are hungry enough between meals (and you will know this because they will actually eat the fruits and vegetables you serve at that time), then offer them a snack.

Follow the weekly instructions listed below until your children eat healthy snacks at snack time and no more than one sweet or unhealthy snack a day. That sweet treat is theirs to control, but make sure it is an age-appropriate serving size. Your children get to decide what the treat will be and when they get to eat it (after lunch).

Start by creating a calendar to track their progress using the "Daily Snack Tracking Tool" at the end of this chapter.

WEEK 1

Replace unhealthy snacks in the morning with a healthy alternative. Your children need a healthy mid-morning snack if there is more than two and half to three hours between breakfast and lunch.

Mid-morning breakfast snacks that will help manage blood sugar levels include a source of protein and either a fruit, a vegetable, or a whole grain. The protein will help settle their blood sugar levels. If your children did not eat fruit at breakfast, make sure they eat some in their morning snack. Try these snack options:

- Almonds (or other nuts) and apple slices
- Yogurt with no more than 23 grams of sugar per 8-oz serving (230 g), or 20 grams of sugar in a 6-oz serving (170 g) (such as Siggi's, Stonyfield, Chobani, Oikos, or Yoplait Greek yogurt) with half a piece of fruit
- Whole-grain crackers and 1 oz (8 g) of low-fat cheese
- Half a sandwich on a small slice of whole-grain bread with nut butter
- Make your own trail mix with ¼ cup (40 g) nuts, 1 cup (225 g) whole-grain cereal, and ¼ cup (35 g) raisins (makes two to four servings)
- Apple slices, celery sticks, or carrots with nut butter spread on them
- Mini muffins made with whole grains
- Mini quiches made in minicupcake tins

WEEK 2

Replace the after-school/afternoon unhealthy snacks with one healthy alternative.

Children need a snack mid-afternoon. These days, kids eat so many unhealthy snacks in the afternoons that they come to dinner full. Limit snacks between lunch and dinner to no later than two hours before dinner or else your child won't be hungry at dinnertime.

Your children can also opt to have their one sweet treat of the day at this time. If they do and are still hungry afterward, offer them a serving of protein to help control the sugar spike (nuts or seeds, a slice of meat, a boiled egg). The best snack option, especially for hungry tweens and teens, is a minimeal (as long as weight is not an issue). Try these snack options for after school:

- Homemade pizzas made on whole-grain English muffins (Note: Most frozen pizza rolls are made with white flour, so look for whole-grain options without sugar.)
- Half a sandwich and veggie sticks
- Hummus, guacamole, or baba ghanoush (a roasted eggplant dip) with whole-grain corn chips
- Fruit and nuts
- Low-fat string cheese with sliced apple
- Veggie sticks spread with sour cream dip, nut butter, hummus, or baba ghanoush
- An age-appropriate portion of the previous night's leftovers
- A minirollup (take a small whole-grain tortilla or a large tortilla cut in half, spread with nut butter, sprinkle on five chocolate chips, roll up, and eat)
- Smoothie (combine ½ cup [115 g] plain yogurt, ½ cup [45 to 75 g] frozen fruit, ½ cup [120 ml] low-fat milk, blend, and drink. You can also freeze it for a frozen treat.)
- Any of the breakfast snacks listed previously.

WEEKS 3 AND 4

Replace after-dinner unhealthy snacking with one healthy alternative or just more dinner. In the next chapter, we will discuss desserts, but for this step we want you to focus on the amount of snacking that occurs after your child leaves the dinner table. For some children, these snacks start within a half hour of dinner being over. If this is the case, it means that your child did not eat enough at dinner. Make sure you don't fall for the "I'm full" ploy that many kids use to get out of eating the healthy stuff at mealtime only to be given lots of nutrient-poor, sweet snacks later. Keep dinner available in the refrigerator to heat up if your children do not eat their meal and pull it out again if they say they are hungry within an hour after dinner. If your children are truly hungry, they will eat their dinner. If not, don't worry; they will eat when they are hungry.

If your children ate an early dinner, they will most likely need a snack before bedtime. If you usually have dessert at dinnertime, your best bet is to separate dessert from dinner and offer it later on. This way, dessert does not seem like a reward for eating dinner and you can make sure that your children eat enough of their meal instead of saving room for dessert. After-dinner snacking can include ½ cup (120 ml) milk or milk alternative to help your child sleep well plus any of the following:

- Whole grains like air-popped popcorn sprinkled with garlic, cinnamon, or another favorite spice
- Whole-grain crackers
- Whole-grain tortilla chips with salsa
- Carrots or celery spread with low-fat cream cheese
- A variety of nuts and slices of fruit
- Edamame (whole soybeans that you can find in the freezer section of the grocery store)
- Dried seaweed chips (it sounds gross, but they are actually very tasty and crunchy—kids love them)
- Fresh fruit salad or cut-up veggie sticks
- Roasted chickpeas with a kick (open a can of chickpeas; wash until bubbles go away; toss in a bowl with 1 tablespoon olive oil, garlic, salt, pepper, and red pepper flakes; spread on a baking tray; and roast at 400°F [200°C], gas mark 6, for 30 minutes)
- Any of the snacks listed previously

The goal is to get your children to eat smaller, more frequent meals and healthy snacks instead of three larger meals: a healthy mid-morning snack if needed, another one after school, and one after dinner. They also have the option to eat their once-a-day sweet treat anytime after lunch.

TIPS TO ENCOURAGE HEALTHY SNACKING

- Leave cut-up fruits and veggies front and center: on the kitchen counter or other high-traffic area in your home.
- Place one serving of your child's sweet treat a day in a baggie and hide the rest.
- Do not have lots of junk food in the house.
- Always have healthy options in the house and car.
- Offer snacks at the same time every day so it becomes routine and your child will be less likely to reach for food willy-nilly in between.
- Have everyone follow the one-treat-a-day rule; children learn by example.
- Cook a healthy snack once a week with your child and make it fun: mini muffins or mini quiches or homemade granola bars, for example.

- Do not offer lots of snacks unless your children have eaten a good portion of their lunch and dinner. You will know whether they have because they will not be hungry within an hour of finishing their meal.
- Avoid situations where snacking is automatic:
  - When your children get home from school, offer a healthy snack and then get them out of the house to play.
  - Set a rule that there is no eating while watching TV; all snacks must be eaten at the table.

- Consider making an exception on Halloween. Let them pick a few of their favorites from their Halloween basket and then buy the rest back from them! A win-win.
- For help, check the "How to Create a Healthy Snack" sheet at the end of the chapter.

Out-of-Control Snacking

Snacking has changed dramatically in the past thirty years. Not only do our kids eat more often, but they also eat more calories. In the 1970s, kids used to get 244 calories from snacks each day. Today, that amount has doubled to 496 calories. To put it in perspective, this extra 252 calories in snacks a day equals the amount of calories needed to gain 26 pounds (13 kg) in one year. This increase would not be a problem if children's total calories consumed every day remained the same and they just ate more calories at snack time and fewer at meals, but this is not the case.

Children's nutritional needs have not changed and neither has our food supply in the past thirty years, so what is causing this increase in snacking?

- Adults have gotten into the habit of offering food to children all the time: before, during, and after school and at playdates, sporting events, group meetings, and so on.
- Children are also being bombarded with messages encouraging consumption of unhealthy food. These messages and advertisements have a big effect on what children eat and how much of it they eat.
- The invention of hyperpalatable (super-tasty) foods makes it hard for your children to say no or stop eating once they start.
- The development of convenient snack packs makes it easy for kids to get junk food not only at the store but also at the gas station, in school, and almost everywhere else they go.

HOW SNACKING INFLUENCES SUGAR ADDICTION

Snacking is where you really see the addictive behavior of sweets come to a head. Sugar addiction and alcohol or drug addiction share these characteristics:

- The craving for more
- Difficulty stopping at one serving; wanting more and more
- Continued consumption despite negative consequences, such as the crash after the high

Because research is in its early stages regarding the addictive quality of food, little has been done to protect our children. What is dangerous is that unlike alcohol or tobacco, children have easy access to foods and beverages high in sugar and the temptation is everywhere they go.

HOW MUCH SNACKING SHOULD MY CHILD DO?

Your child should snack every day. Most authorities agree that it is healthier for children to eat smaller amounts five or six times a day than to eat three larger meals. In addition, individuals with sugar issues also do better eating more frequently.

How much they need to snack and whether or not they need to snack two or three times a day depends on several factors.

1. **The activity level of your child:** The more active children are, the more calories and nutrients they need. An active child needs more snacks than a sedentary child, and your child will need fewer snacks on days that he or she is not very active.

2. **The age of your child:** Young children need to eat three meals and three snacks a day and some older children do as well. Young children have small bellies that cannot hold enough food to supply the amount of calories or nutrients they need between meals. For older children, it is really an individual assessment of how often they need to snack.

3. **The time between meals:** It is not wise for a child with a sugar issue to go much more than two and a half to three hours without eating. By the time children get to the first or second grade, they may be able to go until lunchtime, but it really depends on your child's school schedule.

4. **How much your child eats at mealtime:** If your children do not eat a lot at mealtime, they most likely will need to snack more often in between meals than children who eat a lot at each meal. Children who are natural "grazers" tend to eat less at mealtime and snack more often. As long as they are grazing on healthy food and they do not have a weight issue, there is no problem with this behavior.

5. **How much sugar they currently consume:** Once your children break their addiction to sugar and are no longer eating tons of it, older children may be able to go three to four hours without a snack.

THE BENEFITS OF SNACKING

Children need to snack on the right types of foods for the following reasons:

- Snacking prevents blood sugar highs and lows, thus limiting cravings.
- Healthy snacking provides more opportunities for children to meet their daily requirements for micronutrients, which may diminish cravings as well.
- Snacking on healthy food prevents extreme hunger, and we all know what happens when we get too hungry: we will eat whatever we can find, and lots of it.

The composition of a healthy snack for sugar addicts should include a combination of two items: fruit + protein, or whole grain + protein, or vegetable + protein.

Too much of a good thing, though, isn't healthy, so pay attention to how much your child eats between meals. To figure out whether your child snacks too much between meals, ask yourself the following questions: *Is my child overweight?* If so, it means that he eats too much and/or exercises too little. *Does my child eat his or her meal at lunch and dinner?* If not, perhaps too much snacking is occurring. If she does eat her food at mealtime and asks for a snack in between, then there is no reason not to offer her a healthy snack.

You will also want to look into why your children are snacking if you suspect they snack too much. If you think that your children are snacking because of boredom, stress, or some other emotion, give them something else to do. Have them play outside, ride their bike, go for a walk, dance to the Wii, or participate in any other activity that will get their mind off of food and their bodies out of the kitchen.

SNACKING BASICS

A general rule of thumb is to include a fruit and a vegetable with every meal and at snack time. It is essential for children with a sugar addiction to consume protein at every meal and snack, so add a healthy source of protein to a fruit, vegetable, or whole grain to make a great healthy snack for your child.

Also be aware that when you reduce the amount of snacks that have added sugar or processed grains in your child's diet, they may reach to fruit to get their sugar fix. See the "Fruit Checklist" at the end of the chapter for help. Dried fruit has a lot of sugar, and so do those healthy-looking fruit bars. For example, 1 cup (150 g) of grapes delivers 23 grams of sugar; if you dry those grapes into raisins, 1 cup (150 g) of seedless raisins delivers a whopping 97 grams of sugar. A strawberry 100 percent fruit bar on the market packs 29 grams of sugar while the same weight in pure strawberries has fewer than 2 grams of sugar. A huge difference!

Make sure your child doesn't replace one sugar with another, which is very common, by looking at the daily recommended amounts of fruit that children should be eating (and/or drinking). During this program, allow no more than one and a half times these amounts and limit the amount of dried fruit. Once they have broken their addiction, you can allow more fruit in their diet. See "How Much Fruit Should Children Eat Daily?" in Part II, "The Lowdown on Sugar."

RECOMMENDED DAILY LIMIT OF ADDED SUGARS

The USDA recommends limiting what it used to call "discretionary calories" and now refers to as "empty calories." Empty calories are the calories from solid fats and added sugars. They are called empty because there is little to no nutritional value in them.

Added sugars are "sugars and syrups that are added to foods or beverages when they are processed or prepared," according to the USDA, and we provided a list of them in chapter 3.

Solid fats are fats that are solid at room temperature and they include

- beef fat (tallow, suet)
- butter
- chicken fat
- coconut oil
- cream
- hydrogenated and partially hydrogenated oils
- milk fat
- palm and palm kernel oil
- pork fat (lard)
- shortening
- stick margarine

If your children consume none of the solid fats listed above, which is highly unlikely, especially if they eat baked goods, then all those calories can be used for added sugar. For most children, it is a safe bet to reserve half of those empty calories for added fat and half for added sugar. The following page lists the total amount of empty calories and the amount of added sugar you should set as a daily limit for your child.

USDA Recommendation for Empty Calories and Total Calories per Day*

Age of child	Daily limit of empty calories	Daily limit of added sugar
Children 2 to 3	135 of 1,000 calories	67 calories (4 teaspoons/day = 16 g)
Children 4 to 8	120 of 1,200 to 1,400 calories	60 calories (3¾ teaspoons/day = 15 g)
Boys 9 to 13	160 of 1,800 calories	80 calories (5 teaspoons/day = 20 g)
Boys 14 to 18	265 of 2,200 calories	132 calories (8¼ teaspoons/day = 33 g)
Girls 9 to 13	120 of 1,600 calories	60 calories (3¾ teaspoons/day = 15 g)
Girls 14 to 18	160 of 1,800 calories	80 calories (5 teaspoons/day = 20 g)

*Calories are based on getting 30 minutes or less of moderate activity on most days. Your children may need more or less depending on their activity level. Go to www.choosemyplate.gov/myplate/index.aspx to determine your child's daily calorie requirement.

The amounts listed in the table are a good number to have in mind for monitoring your child's sugar intake and to consider when purchasing food and beverages. If you look at the daily amounts, they do not translate into much when you consider that one 12-ounce (355 ml) can of soda has about 10 teaspoons (40 g) of added sugar in it, a doughnut with crumbles on top can have up to 12 teaspoons (48 g) of sugar, and one cookie can have 1 to 2 teaspoons (4 to 8 g) of sugar. The added sugar in breakfast cereal, fruity yogurt, spaghetti sauce, and other foods also count as empty calories. In fact, some yogurts supply the total daily amount of empty calories listed above for certain age groups—5 teaspoons (20 g) of added sugar per container, according to current food labels.

The Emotional Connection with Sugar

Have you ever wondered what sugar feeds besides the desire for a sweet taste? Childhood is a stressful time for any child, even in the best of families. Children have so much to learn and their bodies grow and change every day. Any changes, even positive changes, are stressful on all of us. Many children reach to sugar to lessen the stress they feel or to deal with unpleasant situations, while some kids eat tons of sugar just because it tastes so darn good and they just can't stop. This addictive quality of sugar and the feeling children get after eating sugar is a way for many kids to soothe themselves. The next time your children want to overeat or reach for sugar, talk to them and spend some time bonding with them. Sugar may just be replacing the good feelings children get when they spend time with and feel loved by mom and dad.

For a sweet option with no sugar, spend time with your child watching a favorite show or movie, or reading a book together, and share air-popped popcorn (add real melted butter), peanuts (in the shell), or another healthy nut.

During this program and beyond, our hope is that you can communicate with your children and learn why they are reaching for the sugar. Is it because they are addicted to the taste, or is there something more going on underneath their eating? Talk to them about their issue with sugar. Children tend to open up more if you are doing something else while you are talking so that the focus is not just on them. You can go for a bike ride, cook a meal together, draw or paint, or take an after-dinner walk while you casually bring up topics. Before you know it, they will be sharing more of their day with you.

You may want to wait until they have gone through the worst of the detox before you attempt to dig into this in any detail because their heightened emotions during this time are not conducive for pleasant conversations. If you feel that there is an underlying issue that you cannot handle, don't resist seeking the help of a pediatric professional who specializes in addiction.

Parent Tips and Tricks

Below are some situations that you may find yourself in while removing unhealthy snacks from your children's diet.

Q: My children get moody, angry, or sneaky when they cannot have the snacks they want. What can I do?

A: Your children's feelings are wrapped up in the food they eat. As we discussed previously, emotions may be a big part of why your children reach for sweet-tasting food. With that understanding, handle your children as you would an addict. Be present for them while they detox from sugar, but give them enough space to vent. Let your children know that it is okay to be mad, but that there are acceptable and unacceptable ways to handle it and give them suggestions: go for a run or bike ride or box it out. This period of intense emotion will not last forever. You will be surprised how quickly they move into a calmer and more centered place, and they will get there faster if they stick to the program. Sneaking treats along the way will just prolong the agony, and you can let them know that.

For children who sneak treats when you are not looking, do not have more than their one sweet treat a day in the house, and make sure all other family members limit their intake of sugar, too. Place one serving of their treat where they have access to it and hide the box for the next day. You can also use the point reward system and remove points each time they sneak an extra treat.

Q: How do I deal with my children when they scream and beg for sweet treats and salty chips at the grocery store?

A: The best way to limit the pleading, whining, and outright screams for products that your children see on the shelves in the grocery store is to try the following tips.

- Give them some control by letting them know that they are in charge of choosing one sweet (or chip) snack item per week. They get to choose whatever they want. Even if you do not agree with their selection, it is important to let your children win this battle. The sense of control they get will help them stick with the program.
- If your children scream for other items in the store, in addition to their one treat, either leave them at home, especially in the beginning, or tell them that they will lose the privilege of picking out their snack for the week. When they scream for more, actually put the item they chose back on the shelf and walk away. You will be surprised how quickly they learn not to misbehave.
- Let your children choose the "fruit of the week" and the "vegetable of the week" to have with their snacks. You can make this a fun experience by investigating new fruits and vegetables online or in books so they get to know the "personality" of the produce. If you have multiple children, let each select his or her winner for the week.
- Before you go shopping, make a list of snacks that your child likes from the list provided in this chapter. Have your child help you find those healthy items when you go shopping.

Q: What do I do about the snacks that are offered at sports games, school, parties, Boy and Girl Scouts, friends' and families' houses, and other kid gatherings?

A: Our kids are offered snacks no matter where they go, and it has gotten out of hand. The best approach when it comes to group events is to work with your child's coach, teacher, or group leader and ask him or her to provide only healthy options. Fruit is sufficient almost every time. If your child needs more than that, it should be the family's responsibility to bring more.

A trip to grandma and grandpa's house can be like visiting Willy Wonka's chocolate factory. Let grandparents know that your children are on a sugar reduction program and why it is so important that they follow the same rules when they are away from home. You can make a list of acceptable snacks and post it on their refrigerator so all they have to do is ask your children to look and see whether what they ask for is on the approved list. This lets grandma off the hook of having to say no and it ensures that everyone is on the same page.

During playdates, let the other parents know that your child is on a restricted diet (if you don't know them well) or that you are limiting his sugar intake (if they are good friends) and ask for their help. You can bring a snack for your child to share with his friend or ask the parents what they will be serving and suggest other options if you know them well. Because birthday parties are planned, let your child enjoy the cake and snacks at the party, but let that be her sweet snack for the day. If she comes home with a goody bag, limit her access to one candy a day as her one sweet treat a day.

If your child receives unhealthy snacks at school, review your child's school nutrition policy. Public schools have a wellness policy that should dictate the types of snacks allowed on school grounds, and private schools have their own set of rules. After discovering what the rules are for your child's school, get involved in changing the policy, if need be, or enforcing it if it is not being followed. The following websites are great resources for changing the food at your child's school to healthy options: www.ruddspark.org, www.angrymoms.org, www.edibleschoolyard.org, www.letsmove.gov/schools, www.healthiergeneration.org/schools.aspx, and www.healthyschoollunches.org/changes/index.cfm.

Q: Our family life is very hectic with after-school sports and other activities. How do I provide a healthy snack when we are all on the go so much?

A: The best thing you can do is to always have healthy snacks in your house or bring them with you when you are on the go. Try these other tactics:

- Children naturally get hungry for dinner around 5 p.m. If it is not possible to feed them at this time, be sure to offer them a healthy snack beforehand instead of letting them graze on junk food.
- Many children have sports schedules that keep them out late at night; divide their dinner in two and serve half in the afternoon and half after they get home.
- Prepare the night before and in the morning before you leave for the day.
- Keep some items in your car that do not rot easily: whole-grain crackers, whole-grain cereal, a huge container of homemade trail mix, whole-grain pretzels, nuts, and small boxes of raisins, for example.
- Keep snack items in one area of the pantry or cupboard and have your children select the items they want for the following day.
- Always have sturdy fruit on hand that does not need to be cut up: bananas, apples, oranges, and grapes travel well. Wash these items when you bring them home from the store so they are always available to your child for snacking. Pears and peaches also work, but wash them the morning of and make sure you don't jostle them because they bruise easily.
- Invest in sturdy food containers, lunch bags, and ice packs that are thick. Fit & Fresh are some of our favorites, and they make lots of kid-friendly and fun items.
- Make a rule before you leave the house that you no longer stop at fast–food drive-throughs for snacks. Make it an occasional treat instead, unless it counts as their one sweet treat a day.

Daily Snack Tracking Tool

Make a calendar, use the one in your home, or download one from the Internet. Offer your children a healthy snack up to three times a day and remember to limit sweet treats to one a day.

Directions: Give 5 points or one sticker (for younger children) each time your children eat a healthy snack and deduct 5 points when they eat an unhealthy snack (exception: the once-a-day-anything-goes-treat).

Week 1: Focus on morning snacks. Replace unhealthy snacks with healthy snacks or start offering a healthy snack if your children are going more than 2½ to 3 hours between meals.

Week 2: Continue with healthy morning snacks. Offer a healthy afternoon snack.

Weeks 3 and 4: Continue with healthy morning snacks. Continue with healthy afternoon snacks. Offer a healthy after-dinner snack if there are more than 3 hours between dinner and bedtime.

The maximum points they can earn is 325.

Made goal: Earned 260 to 325 points.

Second place: Earned 195 to 259 points. Keep following the program until your children earn more points.

Try again: Earned fewer than 195 points: Start the month over again.

I will earn _____ for reaching my goal.

How to Create a Healthy Snack

Create your own snack by following this formula or choose from the list below.

A healthy snack = protein + grain, fruit, or vegetable

Two steps to a healthy snack:

1. Pick a protein

2. Then add a grain, fruit, or vegetable to go with it

Snack time is made easy by asking your child to choose from the list of healthy snacks below. There is even room to add your own favorites.

- Whole grain tortilla chips with salsa + cheese

- Hummus and pita

- Yogurt (preferably Greek) with ½ cup [115 g] or 1 small fruit

- Crackers + cheese + grapes

- Half a sandwich + veggie sticks

- Make your own trail mix with ¼ cup [50 g] nuts, 1 cup [180 g] whole grain cereal, and ¼ cup [38 g] raisins

- Pretzels + cheese + apple

- Low-fat string cheese with sliced apple

- Mini muffins

- Nuts (almonds) + fruit (banana)

- A mini-rollup (take a small, whole grain tortilla or 1 large tortilla cut in half, spread with nut butter, and sprinkle five chocolate chips, roll, and gobble)

- Mini quiches

- Roast chick peas

- Smoothie (combine ½ cup [115 g] plain yogurt, ½ cup [75 g] frozen fruit, ½ cup [120 ml] low-fat milk, and blend and drink. You can also freeze it for a frozen treat.)

List some of your favorite healthy snacks below:

_____

_____

_____

_____

Fruit Checklist

Put a sticker or check mark in the box each time your children eat a whole fruit. For younger children, have them include the color of the fruit or do a simple drawing. Try to stay within your children's daily requirement for fruit.

Age	Daily requirement for fruit	One serving	Two servings	Three servings	Four servings
2 to 3 years	1 cup (150 g) (2 fruit)				
4 to 8 years	1 to 1½ cups (150 to 225 g) (3 fruit)				
9 to 13 years	1½ cup (225 g) (3 fruit)				
Boys 14 to 18 years	2 cups (300 g) (4 fruit)				
Girls 14 to 18 years	1½ cups (225 g) (3 fruit)				

Counts as fruit	Doesn't count as fruit
Whole fruit	Gummy fruit
Unsweetened apple or pear sauce	Sweetened apple sauce or pear sauce
Unsweetened fruit salad	Sweetened fruit cocktail
¼ cup (36 g) dried fruit a day (maximum)	More than ¼ cup (36 g) dried fruit a day
Cut-up fruit packed in fruit juice	Fruit packed in heavy or light syrup
Fruit leather	Fruit-flavored candy

Chapter 5

Step 4:
Make Over Dessert

Set rules and consequences and create healthy, tasty alternatives

Grain-based desserts, such as cake, cookies, pie, pastries, and doughnuts, are the number one source of calories in the diets of children and adults today. What was intended to be an occasional small treat at the end of the meal has become a calorie-laden dietary staple. In reality, there is little to no room left at the end of the day for these extra calories.

Can your children have their cake and eat it, too? Probably not—at least on most nights of the week. Children with sugar addictions need to learn to separate dinner from dessert so that they don't plow through their dinner only to get to the food they really want. They need to focus during meals on eating healthy foods and not "saving room" for pie, ice cream, or cake. The objective is for them to leave the table satisfied and pleasantly full.

Prescription for Making Over Dessert

The goal here is to help you switch from providing unhealthy desserts to yummy-tasting, healthy alternatives while at the same time winning the battle at mealtime.

WEEK 1

Separate dessert—and your child's expectation of it—from dinner. During this week, your goal is to get your child used to dessert not being served at the end of dinner. Have your child leave the table after eating dinner. If your child is hungry within an hour of leaving the table, offer another serving of dinner. If your child gets hungry more than an hour later, offer dessert (if you usually serve it) or a healthy snack (if you don't serve dessert). In this step, dessert is taking the place of your child's after-dinner snack.

In week 2, you will replace the unhealthy dessert with a healthy snack, but in this first, week just serve dessert as usual but serve it *only* when your child gets hungry, an hour or more after dinner.

For those of you who don't serve dessert, skip to week 2 and replace any unhealthy after-dinner snacks with healthy alternatives if you haven't already done so in the previous chapter.

WEEKS 2 TO 4

Begin to eliminate unhealthy desserts on six nights of the week. If your children eat an unhealthy dessert every night of the week, replace one unhealthy dessert with a healthy snack every three days until your children are eating one unhealthy dessert per week and six healthy snacks. This gives you a little over two weeks to make the transition from unhealthy desserts to healthy snacks. Mark off on a calendar when you will be making the reductions and post it on the refrigerator for your children to see and follow along. We have provided instructions for creating a calendar at the end of this chapter. See the "Make Over Dessert Goal Sheet."

If your children eat unhealthy desserts occasionally, reduce the amount of unhealthy desserts by one every three days until they are only eating one unhealthy dessert a week.

If your children do not eat dessert, don't start now. Focus on making sure your children consume healthy snacks between dinner and bedtime if they are hungry or if there are more than three hours between dinner and lights out.

The once-a-week unhealthy dessert is an anything-goes dessert. It can be ice cream, cake, brownies, or one of your child's favorites. Keeping special desserts to once a week teaches your children that dessert is an occasional treat to look forward to, but on most nights of the week they need to eat something healthy. On the anything-goes dessert night, offer only healthy snacks earlier in the day to save those extra calories for dessert.

Post the list provided at the end of the chapter of healthy snack/dessert options that are easy for you or your child to put together. (See "Healthy Dessert Options.") This list puts the decision and control in your child's hands for what to eat after dinner and lets you off the hook for being the dessert police. Feel free to add your own healthy options. Some of the desserts require preparation time; make them in large batches and add to the dessert list for the week.

How to Make Tasty and Healthy Desserts

When deciding on dessert, start by selecting the star of the show: a fruit, whole grain, or dairy. Below are some ideas that are sure to please. We have also provided recipes for items with an asterisk at the end of the chapter.

Starring fruit: Save some of your child's daily fruit servings and offer them as dessert. Have your child select a fruit to focus on each week. It can either be something new or an old favorite. There are many things that you can do with fruit:

- Sliced fruit with or without cheese slices
- Baked fruit*
- Fruit cobbler (homemade, low-sugar versions only)*
- Baked fruit crumble (homemade, low-sugar versions only)*
- Fruit kabobs dipped in yogurt*
- Fruit and chocolate fondue*
- Crushed fruit: pear or applesauce with no added sugar
- Fruit and yogurt parfait*
- Homemade sorbet made with just fruit*

Starring dairy: Serve dairy or a dairy alternative for dessert. Here are some ideas:

- As a special treat, try a new cheese to shake things up so it is not the same old cheese night after night.
- Hot milk with a dash of nutmeg or cinnamon. Have your children create their favorite using spices or other flavorings (with a maximum of 1 teaspoon [4 g] of flavoring that has a sugar base)
- Plain yogurt with or without a crunchy topping, such as granola or nuts
- Homemade frozen yogurt*
- Cheese and whole-grain crackers

- Cottage cheese with fresh cut-up fruit on top
- Low-fat cream cheese on half a whole-grain bagel with 1 teaspoon (7 g) of jam and a sprinkle of dried fruit or 10 chocolate chips

Starring whole grains: To make sure you are serving true whole grains and not an imposter, look for a whole grain as the first item in the ingredients list. Try these ideas:

- Bowl of whole-grain cereal with milk
- Whole-grain fruit muffins with a surprise dollop of jam in the center*
- Whole-grain pancakes with fruit toppings*
- Homemade GORP*
- Whole-grain toast with butter or nut butter and an option of 1 teaspoon of jam
- Bowl of air-popped popcorn with Parmesan cheese or spices*
- Whole-grain crackers with hummus, nut butter, or cream cheese. Have your children be creative. They can make many characters and designs using cut-up veggies and fruits to put on top of the crackers and spread.

The following are other examples of healthy dessert alternatives:
- 1 ounce of dark chocolate; the higher the percentage of cacao solids, the lower the amount of sugar. Try to buy dark chocolate with at least 70 percent cacao solids. If you buy the bite-size miniature chocolate bars from Hershey's, your child can have one with his after-dinner snack, unless, of course, chocolate hypes him up. Look at the sugar per serving on the chocolate and make sure your child does not eat more than 4 grams of sugar; usually that means that you have to decrease the serving size listed on the package.
- A handful of mixed nuts, if allergies are not an issue
- Dessert doesn't have to be sweet: make half a sandwich or any of the snacks listed in the previous chapter.

A Brief History of Dessert

Dessert is sweet for many reasons. From a purely biological perspective, dessert provides no nutritional benefits, and eating too much dessert is considered harmful. Why, then, is dessert so essential for so many of us?

Author Michael Krondl answers this question in his book *Sweet Invention: A History of Dessert*, where he writes, "Dessert is a purely cultural phenomenon." Sweets and desserts were considered a sign of wealth and power in the past, he says, and they are still used today in religious ceremonies, to mark life passages like birthdays, and on other occasions. In the United States, dessert brings with it an image of motherhood: an old-fashioned mother who stays at home and bakes for her family. In addition to the appeal of the sweetness of desserts, it is this archetype of nurturing behind dessert that seduces and calms many of us.

Before the mid-nineteenth century, when industrialization of America's food supply started to replace making desserts from scratch, eating dessert as we know it (cake, pie, and ice cream) used to be only an occasional treat. Sugar was not as readily available as it is today, and it took our mothers hours to make these mouth-watering desserts. Today, with the convenience of hundreds of tasty options at our fingertips, eating dessert every night has replaced what used to take effort and planning.

The environment we live in encourages unhealthy eating: desserts are cheap, tasty, and easy to find. Just take a look at all the mouth-watering varieties of ice cream that are sold not only in the grocery store but also at the gas station, in school, from a truck that drives by our neighborhood, at the pharmacy, and in local specialty shops. Putting a limit on the amount of desserts we feed our children is the only way for them to walk safely through a world full of temptations at every turn.

> We are not going to remove your child's dessert but, rather, encourage you and your child to really enjoy a great dessert once a week.

DESSERT AND YOUR FAMILY'S TRADITIONS

Dessert is an art form with pleasure as its core element, just as with music and any art. This may explain why we react strongly when desserts are removed from our lives. For example, cupcake wars are going on around the country, where school districts no longer allow parents to bring in these mini cakes to celebrate their child's birthday. Many parents react as if their child's basic American rights have been taken away. What is taken away, however, is an easily accessible, affordable pleasure that does not require work for anyone, rich or poor. How many things can we say that about?

We have good news for you, though. We are not going to remove your child's dessert but, rather, encourage you and your child to really enjoy a great dessert once a week.

We appreciate and respect that your personal traditions and cultural heritage are usually wrapped around the desserts you serve. Do you serve a family favorite passed down through the generations? Is it usually sweet or savory? What ingredients do you use and what is the symbolism behind these ingredients? These questions are just some examples of how dessert is more than just the food on your plate.

You may have grown up with fond memories surrounding the desserts you learned to make with your mother or grandmother, or perhaps you shared a dessert tradition with your dad, like learning how to dunk cookies in milk. You do not need to abandon your culture—just make over the desserts you offer now in a way that honors your family's heritage and traditions without making your child sick from all the sugar. If you look back far enough in your family tree you just may find that healthier options were served at the end of the meal: cheese, nuts, and fruit, most likely.

Dessert as a De-stressor

Dessert has become a major de-stressor in our busy lives. After a long day of working and playing hard, going to school, and doing homework, many children like to chill out with a bowl of ice cream or bag of cookies after dinner as a way to calm down, zone out, and not have to think or do anything. Don't we as parents do the same after we put the kids to bed? We finally have some "me time," and many of us zone out with unhealthy food options.

We have done what others (our boss) want or (our kids) need, and now we get to make the decisions; if we want a bowl of ice cream, then by all means no one can tell us we can't. Many times dessert is the big "bug off" to the world where we become childlike in our stance: no one can tell me what to do. We end up hurting ourselves by taking our frustration and bone-tired fatigue out on a bowl of ice cream or chips. Our children do the same, and they probably learn it from watching us.

If you suspect that your children are overwhelmed and eating sugary desserts to cope with the demands of their day, take some time during this step to analyze how many activities and commitments they have on any given day. Ask them whether they think their schedule is too much and problem solve together. Maybe they don't have to do more than one extracurricular activity a season or

> Your children's relationship with food is a cue to how they are dealing with their life.

they can cut back in some other way. Your children's relationship with food is a cue to how they are dealing with their life. It is our job as parents to listen and observe and then step in to take action if their life is not balanced.

REWARDS VERSUS CONSEQUENCES

There are a lot of stories in the popular press and agreement within most of the scientific community that using food as a reward is a bad thing. Research in the 1980s looked at children and adults with eating disorders and discovered that children with militant/authoritarian parents were more likely to develop an eating disorder.

We don't think anyone would disagree that forcing children to eat is not a wise tactic and that it is unhealthy for their long-term relationship with food. Being too strict about food and bringing negative emotions to the table affects your children negatively and should be avoided.

After discovery of the negative impact of having an authoritarian parent, a movement began that gave children too much control over their food choices. The pendulum swung so far in the opposite direction that parents became too lenient with their children about food. Research shows that not only is being too strict unhealthy for your child's relationship with food, but so is being too passive.

Using food as a reward is a catchphrase that many physicians and nutritionists have focused on, often to the detriment of our children. There definitely is a difference between "If you get an A on your test, you can eat ice cream to celebrate" and "Once you finish your healthy meal, you can have some dessert." The first statement is using food as a reward, which we agree does not send a healthy message but a mixed one. The second is an example of establishing consequences as a result of your child's actions and is an essential element in bringing up healthy eaters. It is no more of a reward than, say, getting a good night's sleep after being told to go to bed is.

If we remove rules and consequences at the dining room or kitchen table, we are disempowering a generation of parents, which is exactly what is happening. Our children are sugar addicts because we have allowed it, and we allow it largely because that is what the professionals whom we trust have been telling us to do: we put food in front of our children and then back away.

It is time to set up the rules and follow up with consequences, and to do so in neither a militant nor a passive way. Enforce the rules with a smile on your face and by example (kids can smell hypocrisy a mile away), while letting your children know that the choice is theirs: they can have dessert if they choose to eat their dinner first.

Parent Tips and Tricks

Your child will not like it when you limit desserts and switch to healthy options. Try the following strategies when your child does not eat enough at mealtime or pushes for more dessert:

- Do not let your child (or any other family member) eat dessert mindlessly in front of the television or computer. Make it an occasion to enjoy and focus on without distractions. Haven't you had the experience of eating a bowl of ice cream while watching your favorite TV show and then having no recollection of eating it?
- Give each child one night to be in charge of dessert or snack and let each child take a turn in choosing the week's anything-goes dessert.
- Serve a warm glass of milk at night with their snack or dessert to encourage a good night's sleep. Be careful with serving too much liquid close to bedtime in younger children for whom bedwetting is an issue.
- Research and find recipes together. Involving your children can teach them a thing or two while making dessert.
- They can learn about a new fruit, cheese, or grain when selecting dessert: where it comes from, how it grows, and what are its nutritional properties.
- Have your children discover which desserts are big in their cultural heritage. They can either ask their grandparents or look it up online.
- Discover where a specific dessert originated as a history lesson.
- Discover ways to make favorite desserts a little bit healthier, by reducing the amount of sugar or solid fat, for example.
- For the one anything-goes dessert night, make it on a weekend so that things are not rushed and the extra sugar doesn't hype them up on a school night.

- Dessert time is bonding time: don't lose the opportunity to connect with your child in a fun way. Instead of bonding over sugar, play a game, go for a walk, or bike ride together. If watching a bedtime movie, air-popped popcorn with a bit of real melted butter (not the axle grease used on movie popcorn or in most processed foods) can be a healthy treat (see page 169 for a great recipe tip).

Q: My child won't eat much at dinner but asks for snacks within twenty minutes of being excused from the table and it goes on all night. What do I do about this?

A: Children learn from an early age that if they do not want to eat their meal, all they have to say is "I'm full." Don't take these words at face value but look instead to see whether it's true. "I'm full" is often a ploy that many kids pull to get out of eating the healthy stuff at mealtime only to be given sugary snacks later. It works like a charm because "I'm full" comes with a heavy charge: many parents have been taught not to "force" their children to eat as a backlash to the previous generation's enforcement of the "clean your plate" rule, so as soon as many parents hear these words, they back off immediately.

When small children and toddlers say "I'm full," sometimes they mean exactly that, but just as often they are saying something else they do not have the vocabulary yet to express. "I'm full" may mean I don't like what I'm eating and prefer something else, I'd rather be playing right now, or I just want my dessert and not this broccoli.

As parents, it is our job to discern what they really mean. Look at how much they eat during mealtime and how quickly they ask for a snack or dessert afterward. They should be full enough to last at least an hour after the meal.

Call their bluff by asking whether they would like a cookie, or some other food you know they want, before you let them leave the table. If they say yes, then you can say that they need to finish their meal first. If your child leaves the table but didn't eat her age-appropriate portion, keep dinner available in the refrigerator to heat up later.

Let your children know there won't be any dessert or evening snack until they eat their meal first. Remain calm and matter of fact, and do not engage them when they throw a fit. Keep repeating back to them that the choice to have dessert is theirs—all they have to do is eat their healthy dinner first.

Q: My children plow through dinner to get to dessert. I am afraid that if I take dessert away they won't eat their food.

A: You may encounter some resistance at first from your children when you stop giving them dessert at the end of a meal. One thing that you can do is to not make a big deal when you explain to your children that you are serving dessert later and not at dinner. If your children refuse to eat enough of their dinner, in a calm voice, excuse them from the table with the notice that they are welcome to finish it when they are ready. Do not offer dessert or a snack within two hours of dinner if they do not come back to finish their meal. They may eat little for dinner for two or three nights, but they will soon learn that you mean business and fall into place. After two hours, giving them a healthy snack is fine as long as they do not use this after-dinner snack as an "out" for eating their meal.

In the Kitchen

Here's how to transform sugary desserts into better-for-you tasty treats using healthy substitutions and different sweeteners.

- For most recipes, you can reduce the amount of sugar a recipe calls for by one-third without affecting the quality of the product.
- Add more vanilla extract, nutmeg, or cinnamon to intensify the sweetness of the product.
- Try any of the following sweeteners because you will not have to use as much of them in a recipe to get the same level of sweetness from table sugar. These substitutes may affect the taste of the product that you are baking, but that may be a good thing. Some of these sweeteners also have a lower glycemic index, but that doesn't give you license to overuse these substitutes; moderation is the key for any added sweetener.
  - Honey is sweeter than white sugar, so you do not need as much. Next time you make muffins, use two-thirds to three-fourths the amount of honey that the recipe calls for in sugar and reduce the other liquid ingredients in the recipe by 2 tablespoons (15 g). Baked products sweetened with honey will brown faster, so you may need to experiment with the cooking time and/or temperature; you may need to reduce the temperature by 10 degrees and cook for 5 minutes longer, for example.
  - Use ½ cup (170 g) to ¾ cup (255 g) grade B maple syrup (thicker and less expensive) for every cup (200 g) of sugar called for, and decrease the other liquid ingredients in the recipe by 2 tablespoons (15 g).
  - Use ½ to ¾ cup (120 to 180 ml) juice concentrate for every 1 cup (200 g) of sugar called for in the recipe, and decrease the other liquid ingredients in the recipe by 3 tablespoons (45 ml).
  - Substitute ¾ cup (180 g) raw agave nectar for every 1 cup (200 g) of sugar, and decrease the other liquid ingredients in the recipe by

2 tablespoons (15 g). Agave has a lower glycemic index, which is a good thing, but it is very high in fructose, so make sure your child does not consume a lot of it.

- Try stevia. For every cup (200 g) of sugar that is replaced with 1 teaspoon of liquid or powdered stevia, replace half the bulk that is lost with applesauce, pumpkin puree, yogurt, or another appropriate alternative that would taste good in the recipe.

Make sure you have the following in your kitchen so that you can always whip up a quick and easy dessert:

- Whole-grain mix for pancakes
- Whole-grain muffin mix and/or whole wheat flour
- Cinnamon: not only does it taste good, but it also has been shown to help control blood sugar levels
- Fresh fruit
- Frozen fruit (with no added sugar)
- Sugar substitutes: grade B maple syrup, honey, or agave nectar
- Vanilla bean or vanilla extract
- Unsweetened applesauce or pear sauce
- Raisins or other dried fruit
- Whole-grain crackers
- Popcorn (the kind you air-pop or pop on the stove)
- Low-fat cheese
- Nut butter (check the sugar content)
- Low-sugar granola
- Nuts: pecans, almonds walnuts
- Plain yogurt or vanilla-flavored yogurt (no more than 23 grams of sugar in an 8-ounce [230 g] serving)

Dessert Recipes with a Healthy Twist

WHOLE-GRAIN FRUIT MUFFINS WITH A SURPRISE

Add 1 teaspoon of jam to your favorite whole-grain muffin recipe. Fill the muffin tin halfway with batter, add the jam, and cover with the rest of the batter. Cook and enjoy.

FRIED FRUIT ON WHOLE-GRAIN PANCAKES

Make whole-grain pancakes as directed. In a frying pan, place 1 teaspoon (5 g) of butter, melt over medium heat, and when the butter starts to sizzle, add 1 sliced banana or 1 cubed apple and fry until tender, about 5 minutes. Add a dash of cinnamon, if desired. Top the pancake with the cooked fruit.

TWO-STEP HOMEMADE FROZEN YOGURT

Take 1 cup (230 g) of plain yogurt and add ½ cup (75 g) frozen fruit (raspberries, blueberries, strawberries, peaches, any favorite, or a blend of several). Mix in a blender and serve immediately. Freeze any leftovers. *Serves 1 or 2*

FRUIT KABOBS

Alternate bite-size pieces of fruit on a skewer or toothpick (not for young children, as they may choke on the toothpick). Apples, orange segments, grapes (cut in half for the little ones), bananas, pears, apricots, and berries are all good examples. Watch your children enjoy building their kabobs. They can dip the fruit pieces in a small cup of plain yogurt for extra fun.

FRUIT AND CHOCOLATE FONDUE

For an extra-special treat, cut up bite-size pieces of fruit, melt dark chocolate (1 ounce [35 g] per child), and put in a small bowl. It's as easy as 1 (cut fruit), 2 (melt chocolate), 3 (have a blast dipping fruit in the chocolate).

SILLY-EASY SORBET

Freeze some fruit (banana, peach, berries, or whatever you like), puree in a blender, and *voilà*, you've made sorbet.

FRUIT AND YOGURT PARFAITS

This recipe is very pretty to look at and fun for kids to assemble. You make the parfait by alternating layers of cooked fruit, fresh fruit, granola, and yogurt in a glass.

2 cups (490 g) applesauce (or pear sauce)

1 apple (or pear), cut into bite-size cubes

1 cup (230 g) plain yogurt (not sweetened)

1 cup (225 g) granola

Have your child scoop a layer of applesauce into the bottom of a glass, top with some cubed apple pieces, then add a layer of yogurt, top with granola, and repeat. *Serves 4 to 8*

POPPIN' POPCORN

Popcorn does not have to be boring or plain. You can be as creative as you want and have your children come up with their own recipes. Melt butter and add any of the following: garlic, red pepper flakes, salt, pepper, paprika, chili powder, or *herbes de Provence.* Pour over popped popcorn (that you make on the stove or with an air popper), then sprinkle with Parmesan cheese or ground sesame seeds.

GORP (FOR KIDS OVER AGE FOUR)

GORP is a trail mix used by hikers and stands for "good old raisins and peanuts." Of course, you can vary the mixture according to your children's tastes and preferences.

½ cup (75 g) nuts: almond slices or slivers, pecans, walnuts, or peanuts

   (omit if nut allergies are present)

2 cups (80 g) of one or several whole-grain cereals

   (low in sugar, see the appendix)

¾ cup (110 g) dried fruit: raisins, peaches, apricots, or cranberries

¼ cup (45 g) carob chips or chocolate chips

Preheat the oven to 325°F (170°C), gas mark 3. If using pecans or walnuts, crush them into bite-size pieces (put the nuts in a plastic bag and have your child hit it with a rolling pin a few times). Spread on a baking sheet and roast for 5 to 7 minutes, turning once. Let cool. Combine the cereal, fruit, and carob chips in a medium-size storage container. Add the cooled roasted nuts, and then shake to combine. Give your child ¼ cup (45 g) (young child) or ½ cup (90 g) (older child) for a snack. Let your child choose the fruit, nuts, cereal, and chips to make a different batch each week. *Serves 6 to 10*

BAKED APPLES

This is a tasty dessert, and it meets the fruit requirement as well!

4 apples, cored but unpeeled

2 tablespoons (18 g) toasted nuts: pecans, walnuts, or almonds

   (omit if nut allergies are present)

2 tablespoons (18 g) raisins

¼ teaspoon ground cinnamon

Dash of nutmeg

½ cup (120 ml) apple juice (100 percent juice or cider)

1 tablespoon (14 g) butter or margarine

Preheat the oven to 350°F (180°C), gas mark 4. Place the cored apples in a glass baking dish. Combine the toasted nuts, raisins, cinnamon, and nutmeg. Pack this nut mixture into the cored apple center (kids love to do this part). Pour the apple juice over the apples. Cut the butter into 4 pieces and place in the top of each core. Place aluminum foil over the baking dish and bake for 40 minutes. Remove the foil and bake until the apples are tender 10 or more minutes (test for doneness with a fork), depending on how large the apples are. *Serves 4*

FRUIT COBBLER

This topping is more biscuitlike and less crumbly than the oat crumble.

For Topping:

1 tablespoon sugar

½ teaspoon ground cinnamon

½ cup (65 g) whole-grain wheat flour

¼ cup (60 g) white flour

¼ teaspoon baking soda

¼ teaspoon baking powder

Dash of salt

½ teaspoon lemon zest

2 tablespoons (30 g) cold unsalted butter or margarine

⅓ cup (80 ml) buttermilk

For Fruit Filling:

3 cups (375 g) frozen berries or cherries or a mixture of the two

2 teaspoons (8 g) cornstarch

2 tablespoons (16 g) sugar

1 teaspoon (5 ml) lemon juice

Preheat the oven to 425°F (220°C), gas mark 7.

To make the topping, in a large bowl, combine the sugar, cinnamon, flour, baking soda, baking powder, salt, and lemon zest with a fork or whisk. Cut the butter into small pieces and add to the dry ingredients, crumbling the mixture between your fingers until it is the size of peas. Add the buttermilk and mix just until blended. Do not overmix. Set aside.

For the filling, place the fruit, cornstarch, sugar, and lemon juice in a pan over medium heat and cook until the sugar is dissolved. Pour into a glass pie dish or an 8 × 8-inch (20 × 20 cm) Pyrex dish. Divide the dough into 6 mounds and place on top of the fruit. Bake for 25 minutes. Serve with sour cream or yogurt on top. *Serves 6*

FRUIT OAT CRUMBLE

This dessert can be made with whatever fruit is in season.

For Fruit:

4 to 6 apples (or pears, peaches, apricots, or a mixture of all)

¼ cup (35 g) raisins

1 tablespoon (15 ml) lemon juice

For Topping:

¼ cup (20 g) quick-cooking oats

2 tablespoons (30 g) brown sugar

¼ cup (32 g) whole wheat-flour

¼ cup (35 g) sliced almonds or pecans

3 tablespoons (42 g) cold butter or margarine

Preheat the oven to 375°F (190°C), gas mark 5. Cut the apples into slices, then add the raisins and lemon juice and stir to combine. Place in a greased baking dish until ⅔ to ¾ full. An 8 × 8 inch (20 × 20 cm) Pyrex dish works well. Combine the topping ingredients and scatter evenly over the fruit. Bake for 45 minutes. *Serves 6*

Make Over Dessert Goal Sheet

Make a calendar, use the one in your home, or download one from the Internet.

Directions: Give 5 points or one sticker (for younger children) each time your children leave the table without dessert during week 1 only. During week 2 onward, give them 5 points or a sticker each night they eat a healthy dessert. Deduct 5 points each time your children eat a sweet-filled dessert except for one night a week when it is encouraged.

Week 1: Separate dessert—and your child's expectation of it—from dinner.

Weeks 2 to 4: Begin to eliminate unhealthy desserts on six nights of the week. If your children eat an unhealthy dessert every night of the week, replace one unhealthy dessert with a healthy snack every three days until your children are eating one unhealthy dessert per week and six healthy snacks.

The maximum points they can earn is 100 if they entered week 2 eating an unhealthy dessert every night of the week.

Made goal: Earned 80 to 100 points or 80 to 100 percent of points.

Second place: Earned 60 to 79 points or 60 to 79 percent of points. Keep following the program until your children earn more points and are eating only one unhealthy dessert a week.

Try again: Earned fewer than 60 points or less than 60 percent of points: Continue to replace unhealthy desserts with healthy snacks and desserts until your children are eating only one unhealthy dessert a week.

I will earn _____ for reaching my goal.

Healthy Dessert Options

Try these different healthy options for dessert. We've left room for you to add your own healthy favorites under each section.

Starring fruit:

☐ Fruit and cheese slices   ☐ Pear or apple sauce

☐ Baked fruit   ☐ Fruit and yogurt parfait

☐ Fruit kabobs dipped in yogurt   ☐ Homemade sorbet

☐ Fruit and chocolate

Our favorites:

_____

_____

Starring dairy:

☐ Hot milk with a dash of nutmeg or cinnamon   ☐ Cheese and crackers

☐ Yogurt with or without a crunchy topping   ☐ Bagel and cream cheese

☐ Homemade frozen yogurt

Our favorites:

_____

_____

Starring whole grains:

☐ Cereal with milk   ☐ PB&J on toast

☐ Muffin   ☐ Popcorn

☐ GORP: mixture of nuts, fruit, and whole-grain cereal   ☐ Crackers and dip: hummus, nut butter, or cream cheese

Our favorites:

_____

_____

Chapter 6

Step 5:
Find and Replace
Hidden Sugars

Get rid of sneaky sugar and teach your children to do the same

You have reached the last step of the program and eliminated most of the added sugar in your children's diet. We have already discussed the obvious sources of sugar—beverages, breakfasts, snacks, and desserts—so now we will focus on discovering which foods in your home contain significant amounts of sugar that you never even thought about.

If it comes in a box, bag, can, or bottle, chances are it contains added sugar. This may sound obvious, but you will find added sugars only in processed foods and beverages, not in whole foods from nature.

The sugars in fruits, grains, vegetables, and dairy are part of the plant, grain, or milk. You might think, "Sugar is sugar. What is the difference whether my child gets sugar from a natural source or processed food?" The answer lies with the friends that sugar keeps. The sugar in fruits and vegetables, whole grains, and dairy products keep good company: minerals, vitamins, phytonutrients, and fiber, which are essential for bringing up healthy, strong children.

In contrast, the sugar in processed foods hangs around with the bad guys: trans fats, solid fats, salt, artificial colors and flavors, and preservatives. Avoid or limit these chemicals and nutrients because they can harm your children's health. They are the nutritional equivalent of bullies in the schoolyard.

Follow the prescription below to remove the sources of hidden sugars in your children's diet. Use the "Points Calendar for Tracking Hidden Sugars" at the end of the chapter.

WEEKS 1 AND 2: DROP THE SWEET DIP

Many children love to dip their food into something; to them it is fun and tasty, or it distracts them so that they eat their vegetables and protein. Is there a problem with dipping? Not necessarily. Problems occur when children dip food into sauces loaded with sugar or drench everything they eat in a sauce and therefore never get accustomed to the taste of the real food.

For many children, their favorite dips are often loaded with sugar: ketchup, honey, sweet and sour sauce, and barbecue sauce. Dipping in sugary sauces usually starts by adding ketchup to French fries and then blossoms out of control so that children need a sweet dip with their chicken, eggs, vegetables, and just about everything else. You have probably heard the song "a spoonful of sugar makes the medicine go down"; some kids need that spoonful of sugar to help the healthy food go down, too.

You may think the tradeoff is a good one: eating some sugar to get the vitamins, minerals, and protein that your child needs. By now, you have learned how harmful sugar is and how much "that little bit" adds up. It isn't a good trade, plus your children learn to eat only if there is a sweet taste to their food.

Dipping in sweet sauces is a bad habit that parents have allowed, and it can be reversed or replaced with healthier dips. We have worked with many dippers; one was so addicted to dipping that she had to have ketchup or barbecue sauce with every meal—each piece of protein or vegetable at breakfast, lunch, and dinner needed a dip or she wouldn't eat it. The only things she did not eat with a sweet sauce were candy, cookies, and other junk food.

If your children are dippers, then follow these steps. If they are not, jump to the instructions listed for weeks 3 and 4.

1. Begin by eliminating sweet sauces at breakfast (ketchup on eggs, syrup for sausages, and so on). Give your child three days to get used to that change. Having syrup with waffles or pancakes at breakfast occasionally is fine (no more than once a week), but don't drench the waffles, pancakes, or French toast in syrup. You can also try yogurt or nut butter with fresh fruit as a topping instead of syrup. Offer tabasco sauce or a sugar-free salsa instead.

2. Next, focus on dipping at lunch and either switch from sweet to savory sauces or eliminate the dip altogether. Let enough time go by so that your child gets used to either not dipping or uses a healthy sauce to dip in instead; this should take about three to five days. However, it is fine to serve salad dressing or sour cream with vegetables. Check the Nutrition Facts label and then eliminate all dressings that have sugar as one of the first three ingredients, that have more than 2 grams of sugar per tablespoon, or that contain artificial sweeteners.

3. When your child has made the healthy change at lunch, focus on dinner next and follow the same advice mentioned in the previous step to replace or remove the dips at dinner. Take some time for your child to get accustomed to this step.

Take up to two weeks to eliminate unhealthy dipping or replace with healthy dipping sauces. Healthy dips can include dairy, needed to build strong bones, with chopped-up veggies, plus spices and condiments to give the dip a great taste.

WEEKS 3 AND 4:
FIND THE HIDDEN SUGARS

Look at the *Sugars* content on the Nutrition Facts label of the foods you buy, and start with the foods your child craves. Chances are these foods will contain added sugar. Remember that 4 grams of sugar equals 1 teaspoon of sugar, which is a lot when buying foods that don't need it: crackers, canned vegetables, and sauces, for example.

Your children have an allotment of only an extra 3 to 8 teaspoons (12 to 32 g) of discretionary sugar a day, depending on their age (discussed in the healthy snacking chapter). This small amount of sugar is mostly used up already with their one sweet treat a day, the jam and syrup or cereal they had at breakfast, the yogurt they had at lunch, and any dessert they may have at dinner. To select the best products with the least amount of sugar, follow this advice:

- Look at the Nutrition Facts label and do not buy products that have sugar as one of the first three ingredients (or the top four ingredients if water is included in the top three). Remember to also look for the many names of sugar listed in the breakfast chapter.
- Fat-free usually means the product has more sugar in it than its regular full-fat counterpart.
- Spend time online or at the store looking for varieties of foods that commonly have added sugar in them and select the ones with limited or no added sugar.
- Stay away from artificially sweetened products.
- Take two weeks to switch over your pantry and refrigerator so that you do not have hidden sugars lurking in your kitchen.

The best advice we can give is to feed your family foods that are as close to nature as possible and limit the amount of processed food in your children's diet. For processed foods that can be a part of a healthy diet, such as bread, pasta, rice, and crackers, choose ones that are the lowest in added sugar. Finding the healthiest products is not as easy as it sounds, and we appreciate how difficult it can be to determine the best choices among dozens of options. For instance, choosing a spaghetti sauce can make your head spin if you don't know what to look for. But don't worry; we will teach you how to buy the best products for your family.

What makes shopping for foods low in sugar difficult is the food label. The Nutrition Facts label doesn't show how much sugar is added to a product and how much is there from healthy sources, such as milk and fruit. The added sugar, plus the natural sugars from milk (lactose) and fruit (fructose), are accounted for under *Sugars* on the Nutrition Facts label, so when you are buying a yogurt, for example, you have no idea how much of the sugar listed comes from the milk and fruit in the yogurt and how much comes from added sugar.

We have tried to make it easier for you by listing foods in categories and setting limits on the grams of sugar to look for in a product. Once you compare your children's daily added sugar allotment (just 12 to 32 grams a day, depending on their age as covered in the healthy snacking chapter) to what one serving of pudding, yogurt, or bread has to offer, you or your children will be able to decide whether it is worth it or whether to look for another item with a lower sugar content.

How to Read a Food Label

The only way to stay ahead of the game in the sneaky world of food manufacturing and marketing is to understand how to read a food label. We have provided a "Ten-Point Buying Pocket Guide" to help you flush out hidden sugars and make the best food choices for your family at the end of this chapter.

1. Never, ever pay attention to the front of the box.

Words on the front of the package like "real fruit," "whole grains," "high in protein," and "100 percent vitamin C," are lures to get you to buy the product. Just think of the front of the package as a huge advertisement and not a place to look for the truth. Usually products featuring your child's favorite characters are the worst sugar offenders. Teach your child that cartoon characters belong on TV and not on their food.

2. Determine the serving size before anything else.

The next time you pick up a product and think that it is low in sugar, look at the serving size and the number of servings per container on the top of the Nutrition Facts panel. Five grams of sugar for each serving may sound great, but if you know your child will eat the entire container, and the container has two servings, then the amount of sugar she consumes jumps to 10 grams.

3. Scan the Nutrition Facts label for an overall picture.

On the Nutrition Facts label, carbohydrates are listed as Total Carbohydrate, Dietary Fiber, and Sugars. Although there is a percent daily value (%DV) for the amount of total carbohydrate and fiber, there is no %DV for sugar. A daily value is the targeted amount of the specific nutrient that your child needs to eat every day if your child were eating a 2,000-calorie diet. Because many younger children consume fewer than 2,000 calories in a day, you cannot use the %DV to make sure they are eating enough carbohydrates or fiber, but you can get a sense of whether the product is high or low in these nutrients.

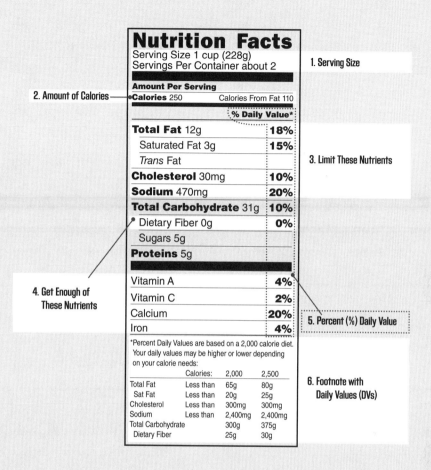

Nutrition Facts

Serving Size 1 cup (228g)
Servings Per Container about 2

1. Serving Size

Amount Per Serving

Calories 250   Calories From Fat 110

2. Amount of Calories

% Daily Value*

	% Daily Value*
Total Fat 12g	**18%**
Saturated Fat 3g	**15%**
Trans Fat	
Cholesterol 30mg	**10%**
Sodium 470mg	**20%**
Total Carbohydrate 31g	**10%**
Dietary Fiber 0g	**0%**
Sugars 5g	
Proteins 5g	
Vitamin A	**4%**
Vitamin C	**2%**
Calcium	**20%**
Iron	**4%**

3. Limit These Nutrients

4. Get Enough of These Nutrients

5. Percent (%) Daily Value

*Percent Daily Values are based on a 2,000 calorie diet.
Your daily values may be higher or lower depending
on your calorie needs:

	Calories:	2,000	2,500
Total Fat	Less than	65g	80g
Sat Fat	Less than	20g	25g
Cholesterol	Less than	300mg	300mg
Sodium	Less than	2,400mg	2,400mg
Total Carbohydrate		300g	375g
Dietary Fiber		25g	30g

6. Footnote with Daily Values (DVs)

4. Look at the fiber content.

Select items with at least 3 grams of fiber per serving if they have more than 80 calories per serving or 2 grams of fiber for items with 80 calories or less per serving.

5. Check the source of the Total Carbohydrate.

Total Carbohydrate = Fiber + Sugars + Other Carbohydrates. Diabetics may need to pay attention to the total carbohydrates that they consume, but if your child does not have this diagnosis, don't worry about the total carbohydrates. Look at the ingredients list to make sure those carbohydrates come from whole grains.

6. Be cautious when looking at the amount of sugars in a product.

Sugars include both the added sugar, which is unhealthy in excess (table sugar or sucrose, and the many other names of sugar listed in the breakfast chapter), and the sugar that is found naturally in fruits (fructose) and milk (lactose). Looking at the sugars listing is a great tool when comparing one cereal to another or one brand of yogurt to another. You will want to choose the cereal, yogurt, or bread with the lowest amount of sugar in it.

- Four grams is easy to remember as a reference point because it is the amount of sugar in 1 teaspoon.
- Because you already know the number of teaspoons of sugar your children are allowed in a day, you can easily determine whether buying that product is worth using up a significant number of their daily discretionary (empty) calories.
- If a product has dairy or fruit, including tomatoes, look in the ingredient list for sugar because you will not be able to tell from the grams of sugars listed how much comes from added sugar.

7. The ingredients list tells you more about the product than anything else on the package.

The first item listed on the ingredients list contributes the most by weight to the product and the last ingredient listed contributes the least to the product.

- If sugar in any of its many forms is listed as any of the first three ingredients, look for a healthier option. Do not count water; if sugar is number four on the list but water is listed before it, then it counts as one of the first three ingredients.
- Buy grain products with the word "whole" as the first ingredient: whole wheat, for example.
- Avoid products with any hydrogenated or partially hydrogenated oil in them.

- Some manufacturers have gotten sneaky and add several forms of sugar. This way, a sugar is not listed in the top three ingredients but takes up several spots below. If this is the case, look at Sugars for the total amount.

8. Buy food in its natural form.

If your children eat 37 grams (¼ cup) of strawberries, they will consume 1.8 grams of sugar, but if they pick up a 100 percent fruit bar in the same 37 gram (1.5 oz) weight, they can eat a whopping 29 grams of sugar. Just because product says "100 percent fruit" does not mean that it provides less sugar than a candy bar. Actually, 37 grams of Twizzlers (4 pieces) packs only half the amount of sugar (15 g) than the 100 percent fruit bar.

9. Avoid products with chemicals.

Some of the unhealthiest foods for your child are those that have lots of chemicals added to them: artificial colors, flavors, and preservatives. Many super-sweet foods contain artificial ingredients, so it is best to avoid or limit them. Go to the Center for Science in the Public Interest's website, www.cspinet.org/reports/chemcuisine.htm#dyes, for more information on the chemicals that may be added to your children's food.

10. Watch out for low-fat and fat-free products.

Low- and fat-free products tend to add sugar to replace the fat, so check the ingredients list. When manufacturers take the fat out of products, they need to add back taste, and most of the time that means they add sugar to fat-free products. It is better for your child to stick to regular-fat options and eat less of them than to go for the fat-free varieties and get the added sugar, unless, of course, your pediatrician has advised otherwise.

Teach Kids How to Shop for Healthy Foods

The ultimate goal in bringing up healthy eaters is to teach them how to make healthy choices themselves by giving them the tools and knowledge they will need. If they are younger, you can ask them to be spies; if they are older, just give them the straight facts if they don't think that being a spy is a cool thing.

SECRET SPY DECODER FACTS

1. Turn the box over. The truth is on the **back of the box**. The front of the box is like an advertisement and doesn't tell the whole truth.

2. Look at the **first three ingredients** in the ingredients list. If sugar is there, put the box back and choose another until you find one that doesn't have sugar as the first, second, or third ingredient. Water doesn't count as an ingredient.

3. Make another choice for grain products if the word "**whole**" is not the first ingredient.

4. If you see a **number** with a color, drop the box fast and no one will get hurt: Blue 1, Blue 2, Red 2, Red 3, Red 40, Green 3, Yellow 5, and Yellow 6. (Also avoid caramel coloring.)

5. **Four** is the magic number, because 4 grams of sugar equals 1 teaspoon. Try to eat foods with 4 grams of sugar or less; a food can have more grams of sugar if it contains dairy or fruit.

6. Avoid foods with ingredients that sound like a list of **chemicals**. If you can't read it, don't eat it!

Sneaky Sugar Categories

The sugar in the following categories counts toward your child's daily sugar allotment (discretionary calories). If your children insist on eating a high-sugar item in the grain or dairy category, it counts as their one sweet treat a day.

CONDIMENTS AND DRESSINGS

When selecting condiments and dressings, always look at the Nutrition Facts label to check for sugar and choose those with no added sugar or fewer than 2 grams per tablespoon. Most fast-food restaurants provide dipping sauces loaded with sugar. Try to avoid those as much as you can; count them as your children's one sweet treat a day if they insist.

Ketchup: Most ketchup delivers 1 teaspoon of sugar (4 g) in every tablespoon. For most brands, the second or third ingredient is sugar.

- Annie's Natural Organic Ketchup has 2 grams of sugar in a tablespoon and Westbrae Natural Vegetarian Unsweetened Ketchup has no sugar added.
- Watch the serving sizes because most kids use more than a tablespoon.
- Try to limit ketchup to just certain items, such as fries, burgers, and hot dogs.
- Mustard and salsa offer healthy alternatives.

Barbecue sauce: Most barbecue sauces have as their first or second ingredient some type of sugar. It's best to make your own sauce so that you can control the amount of sugar your child eats.

Salad dressing: Salad dressings can pack a lot of sugar and brands vary widely in the amount of sugar that 1 tablespoon of dressing delivers: from 0 to a whopping 14 grams of sugar per tablespoon.

- Select dressings that are not typically sweet; avoid honey and French dressings, for example.
- Opt for ranch, vinaigrettes, and other dressings that deliver fewer than 2 grams of sugar per tablespoon serving.

- Newman's Own and Marie's brand of dressings have little to no added sugar in them.
- Try making your own dressing at home with no added sugar.

Mustard: Most mustard does not have added sugar but honey mustards do; many have 2 grams of added sugar per teaspoon.
- Look for mustards with 1 gram of sugar or less per teaspoon: Boar's Head All Natural Honey Mustard has 1 gram of sugar per teaspoon and no artificial coloring, something to look for when selecting mustard.
- Try to get your child used to regular mustard instead of honey mustard.

Salsa: Most salsas have 2 grams of sugar in the standard 2-tablespoon serving size, and for many brands, that sugar comes from the tomato. Salsa can be a very healthy dipping sauce as long as no sugar is added.

Cheese dip: Most cheese dips have no added sugar and are a healthy dipping option, but check the ingredients list to make sure. Some of the more processed varieties of cheese dips like Cheez Whiz have added sugar, so try to make a healthier selection.

Homemade dips: To make a healthy dip, follow these guidelines:
- Start with a healthy base: dairy (cream cheese, yogurt, or sour cream), tomato (salsa), or vegetables (guacamole).
- Fat-free versions of sour cream and cream cheese may add sugar, so select the full-fat versions instead.
- Add your own spices or buy a premade spice mix that has no sugar added.
- Add chopped or pureed veggies to give the dip a nutrition boost.

Beat Sugar Addiction Now for Kids

GRAIN PRODUCTS

Many grain products, such as cookies, cakes, and pies, are loaded with sugar. They are number one on the list for contributing added sugar to a child's diet. We are not going to talk about those products here; instead, we will list the grain products that you might not think have a significant amount of added sugar.

Breads, buns, and rolls: You have already learned how to select whole-grain breakfast products in the breakfast chapter. For breads, buns, and rolls, select varieties with 4 grams of sugars or less for items above 80 calories per serving and 2 grams or less if the serving size is 80 calories or less.

Bread crumbs: Many bread crumbs have sugar as their second ingredient, which makes them an unhealthy choice. Try plain panko bread crumbs because they tend to have little to no added sugar, and then add your own spices, or make your own bread crumbs from low-sugar bread.

Crackers: Whole-grain crackers with no added sugar are healthiest for your child. Look for 0 to 1 gram of sugar per serving.

- Nabisco Triscuit crackers are made with whole grain and have no added sugar.
- Some crackers are made with milk products (whey or milk), which will add sugar; check the ingredients list and select crackers without sugar as one of the top three ingredients.
- Be wary of low-fat crackers because they may be high in sugar.

Granola bars/breakfast bars: Be careful when choosing granola or breakfast bars because they can be loaded with sugar and the amount of total sugars in these products varies widely.

- When making a selection, keep as close to 4 grams of sugar per bar as possible; if the bar has fruit in it, 8 grams of sugar is the limit.
- Annie's has bars with as little as 5 grams of sugar per bar, while Health Valley Multigrain Cereal Bars pack more than 16 grams of sugar in a bar.
- A high-sugar granola or breakfast bar would count as your child's one sweet treat a day.

TOMATO-BASED PRODUCTS

Tomato products are a main source of hidden sugar. It is not possible to tell whether the amount of sugars in a tomato-based product comes from added sugar or the tomatoes. To give you some perspective, if you cooked tomatoes with nothing added or removed, a ½ cup (120 g) would deliver 6 grams of sugar; in comparison, a ½ cup (125 g) of tomato puree packs almost 32 grams of sugar. This is similar to what you learned in the fruit juice section, where manufactures are able to increase the amount of sugar in a glass of juice by adding juice concentrate. The same thing is happening here but with tomato paste. Technically, it is a fruit concentrate, and it enables manufacturers to increase the amount of sugar that spaghetti sauce delivers.

Spaghetti sauce: Tomatoes, plus the carrots or milk ingredients that can be added to spaghetti sauce, contain sugar. If tomato paste is added to the spaghetti sauce, the sugar content goes up significantly.

- Spaghetti sauces range from 2 grams to more than 10 grams of sugar per serving. Your best bet is to look for varieties that do not have sugar as one of the top three ingredients.
- Many brands, from Hunt's to Newman's Own, have sugar as one of the first three ingredients.

- Francesco Rinaldi To Be Healthy pasta sauce, spicy marinara flavor, has 0 grams of sugar and several Classico varieties have 6 grams or less of sugars.
- Look for spaghetti sauce that delivers 8 grams or less of sugar per ½ cup (128 g) of sauce.

Soup: Tomato soups usually have sugar added to them as the second or third ingredient. Below are some examples, but check to make sure that the soups you purchase do not have added sugar in the top three ingredients.
- Campbell's Tomato Soup: sugar is the second ingredient.
- Progresso Vegetable Classics Tomato Basil Soup: sugar is the third ingredient.
- Any soup is suspect, not just tomato-based soups. For example, Lipton Noodle Soup has sugar as the third ingredient.

CANNED PASTA

Choose canned pasta products that do not have sugar listed as one of the first three ingredients. For example, in Campbell's SpaghettiOs (with or without calcium), the third ingredient is sugar.

DAIRY PRODUCTS

In addition to the natural lactose that is present in dairy, many products contain added sugar.

Pudding: Many of us think that puddings are healthy because they provide a lot of calcium. They would be true if they were not loaded with sugar. If you feed your child store-bought puddings, limit them to one a day (it counts as their one-a-day sweet treat). We do not recommend sugar-free varieties because they are just a cocktail of chemicals; many don't even have any milk in them!

Yogurt: Most yogurts are not the great, healthy food that most of us think because many are loaded with sugar: as much as 8 teaspoons in 8 ounces of fruit-flavored low-fat yogurt. It can be a healthy staple in your child's diet, though, if you make the best selections.

- The amount of sugar (lactose) from milk in yogurt ranges from 12 to 15 grams per 8-ounce portion, and that is before any fruit has been added.
- When selecting yogurt, stick to brands that deliver no more than 20 grams of sugars per 6 ounces and 23 grams per 8 ounces. Greek yogurt tends to deliver much less sugar.
- Yogurts in large tubs (32 ounces [907 g]) have more sugar than when packaged in 6-ounce (170 g) cups.
- The following brands delivered fewer than 20 grams per 6-ounce serving:
  - Chobani: most flavors (except strawberry in the 32-ounce container)
  - Stonyfield: fat-free blueberry and strawberry (close at 21 grams)
  - Oikos Greek yogurt
  - Wallaby: low-fat strawberry and the berries (close at 21 grams)
  - Siggi's
  - Yoplait Greek yogurt
  - Fage Greek yogurt: strawberry, cherry, and peach
- Your best bet is to buy plain yogurt and add pureed fruit yourself.
- Do not buy "light" varieties because they have artificial sweeteners in them.
- Count the extra grams of sugar in the yogurt toward your children's daily allotment—to determine the amount of added sugar, subtract the following grams of sugar in the yogurt: 8 grams of sugar for 4-ounce portions, 11 grams of sugar for 6-ounce portions, and 15 grams of sugar for 8-ounce portions.

CANNED FRUITS AND VEGETABLES

If you buy the occasional can of vegetables, choose one with no added sugar. We found added sugar in the following: canned or creamed corn, canned yams, peas, zucchini, and collard greens. Another good reason to ditch the can is that cans are lined with bisphenol A (BPA), and this unhealthy chemical leaches into the food in the can and our children end up ingesting it.

Fruit in a bottle, can, or single-serving cup usually has some form of added sugar: light syrup, heavy syrup, or fruit juice. It is best to avoid fruit sweetened with any kind of syrup. Look for canned fruit with no added sugar or packed in water, and if you can't find any, resort to those sweetened with fruit juice only.

OTHER FOOD ITEMS

Peanut butter: Peanut butter without any added sugar delivers 1 gram of sugar per 2-tablespoon serving. Select those varieties with no added sugar. Most types of peanut butter on the market have sugar as their second ingredient and deliver two to four times that amount in the same serving.

Low-fat and fat-free nut butters have more sugar than regular-fat varieties.

Syrup: Pure maple syrup has less sugar per teaspoon than the blends of syrup that are used in most restaurants and in inexpensive popular brands; use less of the good stuff.

Parent Tips and Tricks

You may run into some common issues when replacing hidden sugars in your child's diet. Learning what to look for and finding the best products takes time, at least in the beginning. Once you find healthy replacements, your child may refuse to eat them. Try the strategies listed below to make it easier for both of you.

Q: My child doesn't like to eat the low-sugar variety granola bar. What can I do?

A: The best thing you can do is put your child in charge. Start by referring to the healthy snacks chapter to determine your child's daily allotment of added sugar. Use a poker chip, marble, or coin to represent each gram of sugar she is allowed and let her put it into a jar to pay for the item she wants.

Let's say your child is eight years old; her daily discretionary sugar amount is 5 teaspoons (or 20 grams). Give your child 20 stickers, poker chips, or dried beans to represent each gram of sugar. At breakfast if she eats a cereal that delivers 8 grams of sugar and a pudding at lunch that has 12 grams, they will have used up all her chips. Once you show your child visually how much it "costs" to stick with her favorite granola bar, sweet sauce, or bread, she may very well say on her own that she doesn't want to waste her sugar coins on that item and decide to eat the healthier, lower sugar variety instead.

Q: I don't have the time to spend looking at all the ingredients lists for added sugar. Isn't there an easier way?

A: We appreciate that it takes time in the beginning to find the healthiest options in each of the food categories. Don't overwhelm yourself on one shopping trip; instead, tackle just a couple of categories during each trip. The next time you go to the grocery store, find the best bread and ketchup; the next time you go, select a healthier crackers and yogurt; and so on. Keep it up until you have removed sources of hidden sugar in your kitchen.

You can also do some of the investigation online. Go to www.peapod.com or another online grocery store and click on a food category. You can look at all the Nutrition Facts labels from home and then go to the store prepared. If your store identifies healthy food and beverages using NuVal scores or Guiding Stars, then it will be much easier because the scientists who developed these food-scoring systems have done the work for you. Don't trust stores' or manufacturers' brands of identifying healthy foods and beverages, such as Smart Choices, Sensible Solutions, and Smart Spot, because the ultimate goal of these industries is to get you to buy more of their products.

Points Calendar for Tracking Hidden Sugars

Make a calendar, use the one in your home, or download one from the Internet, and fill in the weekly goals for your children so that they know what is expected of them.

Directions: During weeks 1 and 2, give your children 5 points or one sticker (for younger children) each time they do not dip their food in unhealthy sweet sauces, such as barbeque sauce, ketchup, and sweet-and-sour sauce. During weeks 3 and 4, give your children 5 points each time they eat a new low-sugar item that you replaced, e.g., low-sugar salad dressing, ketchup, or spaghetti sauce. Deduct 5 points when your children dip their food in unhealthy sweet sauces during weeks 1 and 2.

Week 1 and 2: Stop unhealthy dipping in sweet sauces at breakfast on days 1 through 3, then focus on lunch for days 4 through 8, followed by dinner on days 9 through 13.

Weeks 3 to 4: Find and replace sources of hidden sugars in your kitchen. Switch a sugar-laden item with a low- to no-sugar alternative.

The maximum points children can earn during week 1 and 2 depends on how much and when they dip. If they dip at breakfast, lunch, and dinner, for example, the maximum points earned for not dipping would be 150. Add onto the 150 points another 5 points for each item you need to replace in the kitchen. If your child does not dip in sweet sauces then the maximum points they can earn is 70 in weeks 3 and 4. Add up your children's maximum points and calculate the amount of points they need to fall into each of the categories below:

Made goal: Earned 80 to 100 percent of their points.

Second place: Earned 60 to 79 percent of their points: Keep following the program until your child no longer dips in sweet sauces more than once a week and you have replaced items with hidden sugars from your kitchen.

Try again: Earned less than 60 percent of their points: Keep working on replacing hidden sugars until you have eliminated sugar-laden items from your kitchen and/or your child no longer dips in sweet sauces more than once a week.

I will earn _____ for reaching my goal.

Ten-Point Healthy Foods Buying Pocket Guide

Put this buying guide in your pocket or purse when you go to the grocery store to make shopping for the most nutritional foods easier and faster.

1. Don't pay attention to the front of the box; turn it over for the truth in determining its nutritional value.

2. Determine the serving size before eating.

3. Scan the Nutrition Facts label and look for Daily Value (DV): 5 percent DV or less is low and 20 percent DV or more is high

4. Fiber: Choose products with at least 3 grams of fiber, unless there are fewer than 80 calories per serving; then look for at least 2 grams of fiber.

5. Total carbohydrates = fiber + sugars + other. This information is especially important for diabetics.

6. Naturally occuring sugars include lactose in milk products and fructose in fruit. 4 grams of sugar = 1 teaspoon. To calculate the added sugar, subtract 12 grams of sugar (lactose) from sugars for dairy products. Yogurt: Look for no more than 23 grams of sugar per 8 oz serving, 20 grams sugar in 6 oz serving.

7. Check the list of ingredients: Avoid *hydrogenated* or *partially hydrogenated* oils. Don't buy if sugar is one of the top 3 ingredients. For grains look for "whole" in the first ingredient; e.g., whole wheat.

8. Buy food in its natural form, e.g., whole fruit instead of fruit gummies.

9. Avoid products with chemicals, such as artificial colors, flavors, and preservatives.

10. Watch out for low-fat and fat-free products, as they may be high in added sugar. Look for these names for sugar in the ingredients list: anhydrous dextrose, barley malt, brown rice syrup, cane juice, corn sweetener, corn syrup, corn syrup solids, crystal dextrose, dextrose, fructose, fruit juice concentrates, fruit nectar, glucose, high-fructose corn syrup, honey, lactose, liquid fructose, maltose, malt syrup, maple syrup, molasses, nectars, sucrose, syrup.

Ten-Point Healthy Foods Buying Pocket Guide

1. Look for the **nutritional value on the back of the box**.

2. **Determine the product's serving size** before eating.

3. On the Nutrition Facts label, **5 percent DV (Daily Value) or less is low** and 20 percent DV or more is high.

4. Choose products that contain **at least 3 grams of fiber**.

5. **Total carbohydrates = fiber + sugars + other.**

6. Sugars include lactose (in milk products) and fructose (in fruit). **Subtract 12 grams of sugar (lactose) from sugars for dairy products** for added sugar. In yogurt, look for no more than 23 grams of sugar per 8 oz serving, 20 grams per 6 oz serving.

7. **Don't buy if you see hydrogenated or partially hydrogenated oils** in the list of ingredients or if sugar is one of the top 3 ingredients. Look for whole grains, e.g., whole wheat.

8. **Buy food in its natural form**, e.g., whole fruit instead of fruit gummies.

9. **Avoid products artificial colors, flavors, preservatives, and other chemicals**.

10. **Watch out for low-fat and fat-free products**, as they may be high in added sugar. Look for these names for sugar in the ingredients list: **anhydrous dextrose, barley malt, brown rice syrup, cane juice, corn sweetener, corn syrup, corn syrup solids, crystal dextrose, dextrose, fructose, fruit juice concentrates, fruit nectar, glucose, high-fructose corn syrup, honey, lactose, liquid fructose, maltose, malt syrup, maple syrup, molasses, nectars, sucrose, syrup**.

Conclusion

Where Do You Go from Here?

Tips to continue following a low-sugar diet every day

Congratulations! Your children have completed the five-step Beat Sugar Addiction Now for Kids program and have their sugar intake under control.

If you are feeling a bit anxious, know that it is common and totally natural for you to be somewhat nervous at the end of the program. For many of us, it is easier and feels safer when we are on a prescription and are told what to do. Now that you and your children are on your own, you may wonder whether you can keep it up. We know you can! Why? Because we have not only given you the age-appropriate information you need but also the skills to monitor your children's intake of sugar and reverse it if it starts to creep up again.

Your children's taste buds have become accustomed to a lower "sweet" taste, which means they can appreciate the more subtle sweet aspects of fruit, their blood sugar levels are under control so they will crave sugar less, and enough time has gone by to break the bad habit of reaching for sweets when they are bored, hungry, or anxious. You have taught your children other ways to deal with stress than to reach for food, and hopefully you have grown closer as a family and are "feeding" each other with the love and attention that everyone needs and craves.

We appreciate that life happens, stresses come and go, and our lives pick up pace, sometimes frantically. It is easy to fall back into bad habits, so keep an eye on your children's sugar intake, knowing that this will be where they return to when their lives get crazy. Try and stay as closely as you can to the goals of this program going forward, and if your children's sugar intake rises again, repeat as many steps in this book as is necessary and do it as often as you need to.

Following is a quick review of the main goals of the Beat Sugar Addiction Now for Kids program.

1. Limit juice to 4 ounces (120 ml) of 100 percent fruit juice for children under seven and 8 ounces (235 ml) for those seven years and older each day.

Try and get into the habit of always diluting juice for your entire family. You can save money buying larger containers of juice and it is super easy to add water to these containers to dilute the juice. On days when your child may have more than one juice box because she attended a party, avoid juice the next day and give her whole fruit instead.

2. Use sports drinks only when necessary.

Get into the habit of always having a reusable water bottle on hand and don't buy sports drinks for regular exercise.

3. Avoid or limit (no more than one of any of the following each week) soda, flavored milk, iced tea, or flavored water.

These drinks contribute the most excess sugar in a child's diet. It is easy to slip into "just one more" soda, chocolate milk, or flavored water and before you know it, things have gotten out of hand again. Let them decide where and when to drink their one sweet drink a week.

4. Avoid energy drinks and coffee.

Do not allow your child to consume these drinks for any reason.

5. Stick to healthy whole grains for breakfast with no more than 4 grams of sugar per serving.

Keep breakfast balanced with enough whole grains and protein to start your children's day off right. Once your children have something really sweet for breakfast, they will want more all day and you've lost the battle before their day has begun. On special days where your child has a doughnut or cinnamon roll, count that as his once-a-day sweet treat and go back to eating a healthy

> Once your children have something really sweet for breakfast, they will want more all day and you've lost the battle before their day has begun.

breakfast the day after. You will want to make sure that you provide a healthy source of protein soon after they eat their sweets so that they do not crash and burn mid-morning.

6. Limit sweets to one treat a day after lunch.

Children's diets lack fiber and essential nutrients. Snacks are a great way to get the nutrients your child needs. Try and provide the basic essentials at snack time: fruit, vegetables, whole grains, and low-fat dairy foods, and limit sweet treats to one a day.

7. Limit desserts to one anything-goes dessert each week.

Plan ahead for the week's special dessert. If you know that there is a party or that you will be going out one night, save the dessert for that special occasion.

8. Avoid dipping in sweet sauces.

Don't start this habit because you think it is the only way to get your children to eat the healthy stuff. You are training their taste buds to want more sweets and making it harder for your children to control their sugar intake overall.

9. Remove sources of hidden sugar from your kitchen.

Spend some time to discover healthy foods low in added sugar, plus condiments that your children will eat. Look at the label every now and again because recipes change from time to time and manufactures may sneak sugar into a product that didn't have any before. Watch your children and if you see them having a hard time limiting a certain food, then look at the ingredients list for added sugars. Children who crave sugar tend to ferret it out in unexpected places.

Here are some other suggestions to help your child maintain the healthy changes that were made during the Beat Sugar Addiction Now for Kids program.

- Don't worry about the amount of fruit you child eats as long as it is in reasonable limits (no more than twice the recommended amount of fruit and not if the excess displaces other healthy foods like vegetables) and make sure you focus on whole fruit instead of dried fruit. As you have learned, once you remove the water from fruit the amount of sugar increases dramatically and a small amount of dried fruit packs a lot of sugar in one serving.

- If you are concerned about being that family that no kids want to visit because you don't serve soda, chips, and candy, make it fun some other way. Bake homemade whole-grain cookies, have kids dip fruit in chocolate, offer great-tasting popcorn. You can still have fun and be healthy. Many families no longer bake from scratch; have fun with your children and their friends by making something homemade.

- Every month or so, pay attention to the amount of sugar-sweetened drinks, treats, and desserts that your children consume to make sure they continue to consume a diet low in added sugars.

- You can always keep a chart that monitors your children's intake of sugar-sweetened foods as long as you think it is needed. Have your children put a mark or sticker each time they consume a sweet food or drink.
- Stick as closely as you can to the goals. We know that some months, especially those packed with holidays, are tough. On days that there is excess sugar consumption, up the exercise and avoid sugar the next day.
- Have your children sign the "Maintenance Sugar Pledge" provided at the end of the chapter. It will serve as a friendly reminder if their sugar intake starts to creep up again.
- Reward your children (and yourself!) for a job well done with something other than food, of course! Use the "Total Points Calculation for BSAN for Kids Program" at the end of the chapter to track your children's progress and keep them motivated.

It has been our pleasure taking you through this five-step journey. We wish you and your children the best: a long, happy, and healthy life full of the sweetest treasure of all—time together enjoying one another.

Sugar Maintenance Pledge

Sit down with your children and discuss the following list together when they have completed the program. Have your children initial each of the following agreements after you discuss it with them.

I, _____, promise to do my best to limit sugar in my diet.
I understand that too much sugar is harmful to my body and I agree to the following:

- I will drink water, plain milk, and 100 percent juice every day and save soda, flavored milk, and other sweetened drinks for a special treat that I can have once a _____ (week/month).

- I will not drink energy drinks because they can harm my body.

- I will eat healthy whole grains for breakfast and limit doughnuts, cinnamon buns, pastries, and other sugary foods to _____ (fill in mutually agreed upon amounts, e.g., one per/month or one per week for any of them, not one of each and they will count as the once a day sweet treat).

- I get to choose the healthy snacks that I want to eat every day.

- I will limit sweet treats to one a day and if I eat more than one sweet treat a day, I understand that I will get no sweet treats the next day.

- I will limit dipping in ketchup or other sweet sauces to the following foods: _____, _____, _____

Once a week, I will enjoy a great dessert and on the other nights I agree to eat a healthy dessert. I choose health!

_____   _____
Signature of child   Signature of parent

Total Points Calculation for BSAN for Kids Program

Keep track of your children's progress so that you and they can keep motivated! Choose a grand prize together and fill in the chart at the beginning and end of each step. Make sure to praise them for the points they earned and to keep it up.

Step	Maximum points (A)	Points earned (B)
Limit juice		
Replace flavored milk		
Eliminate soda and energy drinks		
Replace flavored water and sports drinks		
Avoid coffee and caffeinated tea		
Revamp breakfast		
Healthy snacking		
Healthy desserts		
Find and replace hidden sugars		
TOTAL		

Step 1: Add up the maximum points that could have been earned (column A)

Step 2: Add up the points your child earned in each step (column B)

Step 3: Divide total in column B (your child's points) by total in column A (maximum points)

Step 4: Multiply this number by 100

Step 5: Determine which prize your child earned:

Tier 1 prize (80 to 100 percent points) _____
(fill in prize)

Tier 2 prize (60 to 79 percent points) _____
(fill in prize)

Tier 3 (fewer than 60 percent points). Try again.

I will earn _____ for reaching my goal.

Resources

Introduction

The *A.D.D. Nutrition Solution: A Drug-Free 30-Day Plan* by Marcia Zimmerman, M.Ed., C.N.

Beat Sugar Addiction Now! by Jacob Teitelbaum, MD, and Chrystle Fiedler

USDA *Dietary Guidelines for Americans*, 2010, www.cnpp.usda.gov/dietaryguidelines.htm

Yale Rudd Center for Food Policy & Obesity: Food & Addiction, www.yaleruddcenter.org/what_we_do.aspx?id=262

Chapter 1

The Discipline Book: How to Have a Better-Behaved Child from Birth to Age Ten by Martha Sears and William Sears

Positive Discipline for Teenagers by Jane Nelsen, EdD, and Lynn Lott

Chapter 2, Part I

Dietary Reference Intakes: The Essential Guide to Nutrient Requirements (Washington, DC: The National Academies Press, 2006), pp. 156–166.

Harvard School of Public Health: The Nutrition Source: Healthy Drinks, www.hsph.harvard.edu/nutritionsource/healthy-drinks

Kid's Health from Nemours: Healthy Drinks for Kids, http://kidshealth.org/parent/nutrition_center/healthy_eating/drink_healthy.html

Chapter 2, Part II

Sweet Deception: Why Splenda, NutraSweet, and the FDA May Be Hazardous to Your Health by Joseph Mercola and Kendra Degen Pearsall

Whitewash: The Disturbing Truth About Cow's Milk and Your Health by Joseph Keon and John Robbins

"Clinical Report—Sports Drinks and Energy Drinks for Children and Adolescents: Are They Appropriate?"
http://pediatrics.aappublications.org/content/early/2011/05/25/peds.2011-0965.full.pdf+html

The American Academy of Pediatrics: The Use and Misuse of Fruit Juice in Pediatrics, http://aappolicy.aappublications.org/cgi/reprint/pediatrics;107/5/1210.pdf

Kid's Health from Nemours: Caffeine and Your Child,
http://kidshealth.org/parent/growth/feeding/child_caffeine.html

Kid's Health from Nemours: Sports and Energy Drinks, http://kidshealth.org/parent/sports_medicine_center/q_a/power_drinks.html

The National Dairy Council, www.nationaldairycouncil.org

Stevia www.truvia.com

SweetLeaf www.sweetleaf.com

Chapter 3

Glycemic Index Cookbook for Dummies by Rosanne Rust and Meri Raffetto

Build Healthy Kids: Choosing Healthy Food, www.buildhealthykids.com/choosinghealthy.html

Epicurious: Cooking with Healthy Whole Grains, www.epicurious.com/articles guides/healthy/nutritiousdishes/grains

Harvard School of Public Health: The Nutrition Source: Protein,
www.hsph.harvard.edu/nutritionsource/what-should-you-eat/protein

Kid's Health from Nemours: Hypoglycemia
http://kidshealth.org/parent/diabetes_center/diabetes_basics/hypoglycemia.html

Kid's Health from Nemours: Type 2 Diabetes: What Is It?
http://kidshealth.org/parent/medical/endocrine/type2.html

The Whole Grain Council, www.wholegrainscouncil.org

Chapter 4

The Family Nutrition Book: Everything You Need to Know About Feeding Your Children—From Birth through Adolescence by William Sears

Build Healthy Kids: Limit Treats, www.buildhealthykids.com/take12snacks.html

www.ChooseMyPlate.gov: What Are Empty Calories?
www.choosemyplate.gov/weight-management-calories/calories/empty-calories.html

www.ChooseMyPlate.gov: *Empty Calories—How Do I Count the Empty Calories I Eat?*
www.choosemyplate.gov/food-groups/emptycalories_count_table.html

Healthy Children: Snacking and Grazing, www.healthychildren.org

Fit and Fresh Products, www.fit-fresh.com

Chapter 5

Beat Sugar Addiction Now! Cookbook: Recipes That Cure Your Type of Sugar Addiction and Help You Lose Weight and Feel Great! by Jacob Teitelbaum, MD, Deirdre Rawlings, and Chrystle Fiedler

Sweet Invention: A History of Dessert by Michael Krondl

www.AllRecipes.com: *Baking with Sugar and Sugar Substitutes,* http://allrecipes. com/howto/baking-with-sugar-and-sugar-substitutes (Note: Don't use the sugar substitutes mentioned.)

Nutrition and Healthy Eating: Recipe Makeovers: 5 Ways to Create Healthy Recipes, www.mayoclinic.com/health/healthy-recipes/NU00584

Chapter 6

Guiding Stars
http://guidingstars.com

Harvard School of Public Health: The Nutrition Source: How to Spot Added Sugar on Food Labels, www.hsph.harvard.edu/nutritionsource/healthy-drinks/added-sugar-on-food-labels

NuVal, www.nuval.com

U.S. Food and Drug Administration: The Food Label and You—Video, www.fda.gov/Food/ResourcesForYou/Consumers/NFLPM/ucm275409.htm

U.S. Food and Drug Administration: Nutrition Facts Label: Programs and Materials, www.fda.gov/Food/ResourcesForYou/Consumers/NFLPM/default.htm

Conclusion

Dr. Deborah Kennedy

www.buildhealthykids.com/blog

Dr. Jacob Teitelbaum

www.endfatigue.com

Programs of Note

Build Healthy Kids

Drdeb@buildhealthykids.com

www.buildhealthykids.com

Build Healthy Kids is a step-by-step guide for parents who want to bring up healthy and active children. It focuses on twelve national nutrition and exercise recommendations, one each month. Each of the twelve building blocks is based on the current recommendations of the American Academy of Pediatrics, the American Heart Association, and the USDA *Dietary Guidelines for Americans*, 2010. Parents start with a free assessment to see how well their child is meeting national requirements for nutrition and exercise and then they follow the Build Healthy Kids program, which focuses on making one change a month.

The NutriBee^{sm} National Nutrition Competition
www.admin@nutribee.org
www.NutriBee.org

The National Nutrition Bee and the National Nutrition Bowl, known as the NutriBee and the NutriBowl Team competitions, are unique nutrition education concepts. This new program is currently being developed by Ingrid Kohlstadt, MD, MPH, a physician and nutrition specialist who is an associate at The Johns Hopkins Bloomberg School of Public Health.

The NutriBee and NutriBowl National Nutrition Competitions empower students to learn about nutrition. The programs combine entertainment and education to form a quiz-show-style competition for fifth- and sixth-graders. The mission of these competitions is to engage and educate children about nutrition's relationship to good health in a fun, motivational, and competitive hi-tech venue with the contestants working individually in the NutriBee, and together in teams for the NutriBowl. Prizes for winning finalists will include scholarships, awards, travel, and national recognition.

Acknowledgments

JT: So many special people helped make this book possible that I cannot possibly list them all. In truth, I have created nothing new; I have simply synthesized the wonderful work done by an army of hardworking and courageous physicians and healers.

I would like to extend my sincerest thanks to the following people:

First and foremost, my wife Laurie, for her patience with me during the writing of this book.

My mom and dad, who continue to inspire me despite having passed on long ago.

My staff, especially Cheryl Alberto, who keep everything handled while I'm busy writing and teaching. Their hard work, compassion, and dedication (and, I must admit, patience with me) are what make my work possible.

My wonderful, amazing, and dedicated publicist and friend, Dean Draznin, and his staff, who are my teammates in making effective treatment and health available to everyone. A special thanks also to Richard Crouse and Rich Mendelson, my computer "genies." Whenever I just wish for stuff, they make it happen!

The Anne Arundel Medical Center librarian, Joyce Miller. Over the past thirty years, I have often wondered when she would politely tell me to stop asking for so many studies. So far, she has not. In fact, she always smiles when I ask her for more.

Bren Jacobson and Dr. Alan Weiss, who keep me intellectually, emotionally, and spiritually honest while reminding me to reclaim my sense of humor.

I would especially like to thank Dr. Deb, who taught me so much as we worked together on this book, and Chrystie Fiedler who inspired the BSAN series.

And to the Fair Winds Press team, including Jill Alexander, Cara Connors, John Gettings, Will Kiester, and our agent, Marilyn Allen.

DK: Being a huge sugar addict as a child gave me special insight while writing this book. It is something I control, most of the time, to this day. I could not have written this book if it weren't for the multitude of children whom I have had the pleasure of working with, playing with, and observing throughout my many years of practicing as a nutritionist. To the kids who blessed my day at the Integrative Therapies Program for Children with Cancer to the little tykes who joined my Build Healthy Kids class, you all taught me each and every day. I had the honor of learning from these angels. How lucky am I!

I have thoroughly enjoyed writing this book with Jacob Teitelbaum and the staff at Fair Winds Press. Jill Alexander and Cara Connors were a delight to work with, and a special thanks to my agent, Marilyn Allen of the Allen O'Shea Literary Agency.

The support of my family makes it all possible, for without their encouragement and help, I could not have found the time to do what I love—write books!

About the Authors

Jacob Teitelbaum, MD, is an internal medicine specialist who has treated sugar-related issues, including chronic fatigue syndrome and pain, for more than thirty years. He is medical director of the national Fibromyalgia and Fatigue Centers (www.fibroandfatigue.com) and author of the popular free iPhone app Cures A–Z. He is the coauthor of *Beat Sugar Addiction Now!* and *Beat Sugar Addiction Now! Cookbook.*

He is the senior author of the landmark studies "Effective Treatment of Chronic Fatigue Syndrome and Fibromyalgia—a Randomized, Double-Blind, Placebo-Controlled Intent to Treat Study," "Effective Treatment of Chronic Fatigue Syndrome, Fibromyalgia with D-Ribose (Corvalen): A Multicenter Study," "Effective Treatment of Autism with NAET," and the best-selling book *From Fatigued to Fantastic!* and *Pain Free 1-2-3—A Proven Program for Eliminating Chronic Pain Now!* (McGraw-Hill). He does frequent media appearances on *Good Morning America*, CNN, Fox News Channel, *The Dr. Oz Show*, and *Oprah & Friends* with Dr. Mehmet Oz. He lives in Kona, Hawaii. His website is www.vitality101.com.

Deborah Kennedy, PhD, is a pediatric nutritionist with twenty-five years of experience in the field of nutrition. She currently has a patent pending for a healthy meal delivery system and is the CEO and founder of www.BuildHealthyKids.com. She was the associate director of nutrition at Yale's Prevention Research Center, where she helped develop the Overall Nutritional Quality Index (ONQI), which went on to score foods for NuVal. She has created nonprofit organizations, including Turn the Tide Foundation for Dr. David Katz, which focuses on childhood obesity, and Foundation for the Advancement of Cardiac Therapies (FACT) for Dr. Mehmet Oz. She is the mom of two young boys and is passionate about the health of not just her children but all children everywhere.

Index

Beat Sugar Addiction Now for Kids